PATIENT ADVOCACY MATTERS II

Protection of your Rights as a patient
In the new world Of U.S. Healthcare

With Edmund G. Turner

NSHORE ✓ PUBLISHING

Chicago, Illinois

NSHORE ✓ PUBLISHING
Chicago, Illinois

150 S. Wacker Dr. Ste 2400, Chicago, IL 60606
www.northshoreRN.com

Patient Advocacy Matters © 2016 by NShore Publishing
An Imprint of Dreher Publishing in association with
Quintessential Publishing, LLC
ISBN: 978-0692078792

Library of Congress Control Number:
2091894873

Edited by Edmund G. Turner

Cover designed by Danijela Mijailovic

Manufactured and Printed in the United States of America

Dedication

Dedicated to our family's Papa, our loving and wise patriarch, counselor, supporter, and role model in all matters of business and financial management. You are the greatest curmudgeon of all and I love you in spite of it; what would we do without you?

Thanks most of all for teaching me, a seasoned career ICU nurse, how to advocate for my own family. I never realized how powerful that role could be until your critical illness off the coast of Belize in 2008.

Contents

Acknowledgments

This project has been a labor of love for me, as I genuinely want to help as many people as possible take charge of their health by becoming their own best advocate. If the patient is unable to effectively self-advocate, I pray they find someone who is armed with the knowledge I share in this book.

I'd like to thank my editor, Edmund G. Turner, for the wise suggestions in this second edition of Patient Advocacy Matters. Healthcare is changing so quickly that multiple additions, some deletions, and many new stories have been added for the benefit of readers and healthcare consumers from a wide variety of backgrounds. We hope that these changes will add value and prevent more harm to patients everywhere.

My husband Dean, who is my best friend and supporter, believed in my talent and abilities for longer than anyone, and saw them firsthand when his father was in the midst of a medical crisis. His father, Ed, was the inspiration for my career change, and his mother, Ramona, has been my unwavering champion and supporter, undoubtedly telling all her bridge partners today to buy this book.

I am enormously grateful to my former nurse manager Sharon Dmitrijevich who saw something more in me many years ago and encouraged me to pursue a career in patient advocacy. To Karen Mercereau of RN Patient Advocates, who wrote the foreword of this book, I will be forever grateful for equipping me to make a career out of my passion through her intensive and thorough training curriculum for nurse advocates in Arizona. She has been my champion and supporter since my career in advocacy began.

To my dear friends and colleagues Kate Curler, Carrie Espinoza, Jean Lyon, and Danny McLane, who contributed their own stories and wisdom to this book, I am forever in your debt.

You all helped me push through to ensure that we finished this project with a bang. I am elated to have such a supportive community of family, friends, peers and associates who join me on this journey to true patient advocacy.

Foreword *(by Karen Mercereau, RN)*

When I walk into an attorney's office to negotiate and read a contract, I get anxious because I do not speak legalese. I am uncomfortable participating in activities that absolutely affect my life while I cannot comprehend what is happening and what I need to do. Mistakes happen all too often and they can cause real harm.

Welcome to Healthcare 101.

Do you know your rights? Do you understand *all* the ramifications of your medications and treatment plan? Are you aware that the health insurance industry is dictating what can happen to you and what your physician must do in order to be reimbursed?

The stream of research and information in medicine today is at a feverish pitch; but do *you* understand that you really do have choices—if only you understood what they are? Do you realize that you absolutely can say, "No, not until I understand this better"?

The latest study on the number of misdiagnoses in the US by the Institute of Medicine (2015) reported that there are 12 million misdiagnoses each year. Why? Does this mean that our doctors and nurses have suddenly become substandard?

No.

A couple of factors create this storm. First, the insurance industry dictates production quotas for healthcare providers, so everyone is in a very big hurry—all the time. Reimbursement is tied to levels of "production." This is a recipe for error and missed opportunities.

Secondly, many preventable medical errors occur due to lack of accurate medical histories; and unfortunately, it doesn't matter if the records are electronic or paper. They are usually not connected. An example? A patient with a history of renal dysfunction is experiencing severe pain. He arrives in the ER with a companion who is very upset and does not know what to tell the medical staff other than the history of the current issues. The patient is sent to have some radiology work done and a dye, or contrast, is administered in order to see more detail during the test. The patient's kidneys stop working properly due to the contrast chemicals. If the physician had known about the patient's kidney history, this outcome could have been avoided. Lack of contextual medical history leads to hundreds of thousands of preventable medical errors, many of them fatal.

Dr. John T. James, a toxicologist at NASA, published the results of a national study in 2013 that investigated the number of preventable medical errors that contributed to a patient's death. Better sit down now.

Between 220,000 and 440,000 deaths due, at least in part, to preventable medical error occur every year! This was published in the Journal of Patient Safety in 2013. What if you do not know the proper questions to ask? (By the way, this number is derived from only the hospitalized population, not the whole population.)

Speaking of asking questions, it is surprising to note that the only major national groundbreaking study on health literacy was published by the Department of Health and Human Services. The National Assessment of Adult Literacy completed a study in 2003 that uncovered a startling fact: "Only 12 percent of U.S. adults had proficient health literacy. Over a third of U.S. adults—77 million people—would have difficulty with common health tasks, such as following directions on a prescription drug label..."

Do *you* know the right questions to ask?

These studies represent part of the context in which the field of patient advocacy has developed. Independent, RN-based patient advocacy, the most clinically in-depth form of patient advocacy, has delivered patient advocacy care across the US since 2002.

Teri Dreher, RN, iRNPA (independent RN Patient Advocate) is one of the pioneers of this necessary and valuable service. The picture Mrs. Dreher paints through the stories and facts in this eye-opening book is a picture all too familiar to millions of Americans. You will most likely see yourself or one of your loved ones reflected in the information presented here. Let Teri help you to understand how you can become an active participant and advocate in your own healthcare—the information in this book can save your life.

– Karen Mercereau, RN, iRNPA

Founder RN Patient Advocates, PLLC, 2002

Creator of the RN Patient Advocacy Process

How It All Began
The Birth of an RN Patient Advocate

Before I begin the story of the medical crisis that changed my life forever, I'd like to share a brief life history of my beloved father-in-law (whom we lovingly refer to as Papa), the man whose catastrophic health crisis catapulted me into the profession of healthcare advocacy. Papa loves his family dearly and has demonstrated that to all of us in countless ways over the years (I think I may actually have fallen in love with my in-laws before I did my husband!). Papa is a very outgoing, likable guy who makes everyone feel welcome and cared about. He was one of eight children who grew up in a poor farming community in Wisconsin. Since he was a child during the Great Depression, he experienced extreme poverty firsthand. His father used to bring roadkill home for dinner and from early on, he and his brothers knew the value of hard physical labor. Papa grew up with lofty dreams of making it out of that little community and making something of himself. His childhood sweetheart Ramona, whom we call Nanny, shared that dream—so they moved to the big city: Madison, Wisconsin. While in Madison, Papa attended night school while he worked two jobs to support his young family. He worked incredibly hard and eventually became head of the tax department at Baxter Healthcare in northern Illinois; later he left that job to start his own accounting firm in his new hometown of Libertyville, Illinois. He was not just any accountant; he was well respected in his field and a community leader. He enjoyed a lucrative career and invested wisely. All of his friends and clients respected him and agreed that his life was not too shabby for a small-town Wisconsin farm boy.

Education was a core family value to both Papa and Nanny, and once Papa received his accounting degree, he set the goal of one day paying for every one of his children to get the best education possible. Later in his career, Papa's generous and loving spirit, combined with his outstanding abilities as an accountant, allowed him also to provide every grandchild with higher education. We can never thank Papa enough for his love and sacrifice in providing for his family's education.

Papa is a wise man. He has taught all of us that there are no do-overs with family, and he has demonstrated through his actions the true meaning of loyalty to one's family. At the height of his career, his beloved Ramona was diagnosed with a particularly aggressive form of lung cancer. Upon learning of the diagnosis, Papa put the brakes on his career. His life priorities changed in a heartbeat and he dedicated the rest of his life to his family. He sold his accounting business and stayed by Ramona's, Nanny's, side through an arduous course of extensive surgery, radiation, and chemotherapy that ultimately cured her disease. Even though it has left her with a partial right arm paralysis and chronic pain, we are so grateful that Nanny is considered cured of her cancer. We are grateful for them both and consider them both precious to our entire family.

CHAPTER 1
Modern Healthcare and My Inspiration for Advocacy

Patient advocacy is who I am and what I do. I am a voice for people without a voice, and I absolutely love using my decades of intensive care experience to help save people's lives outside the hospital like I did for so many years within the boundaries of the ICU. Though my present career path is not nearly as lucrative as my former one, I must say that this is the greatest and best career decision of my life. The intangibles are priceless. Patient advocates make a difference, every day, whether they are medically trained or not. Today, everyone needs a patient advocate!

Some call it private professional healthcare advocacy, patient navigation, or a variety of other names. The model I discuss here is the model of privately paid professionals who do not work for an institution or an insurance company.

The lines of allegiance are clear when the patient pays for services. We do not work for the hospital. We do not work for the doctors. We do not work for insurance companies. We are *private* patient advocates, hired by patients and their families to protect patient rights and to avoid medical error. We advocate for patients by–in extreme cases–helping to save their lives. As advocates for the patient, we also help patients to save money and most of all, we help save frustration for all who are struggling with modern healthcare.

Some of us have medical or nursing backgrounds, some are social workers, geriatric care managers and lay people who have studied the system well. We know how to come alongside patients and ensure they have better communication with healthcare providers. A big part of better communication with healthcare providers can be as simple as more education. More education on the patient's part, empowers them as well; this helps to protect them and improves their safety as they navigate through life's medical challenges.

Modern healthcare is complex and frightening for many, and those who choose to hire their own advocate will almost always tell you that it is one of the best decisions they ever made. But consumers need to know that this is a fairly new field; it's only about a decade old, and there is no national accreditation process in place yet. Right now, that's the biggest challenge for leaders in this industry: to develop a test that will certify competency for both medical and non-medical advocates. Not everyone needs a nurse or doctor to be their advocate. The level of medical complexity depends on the necessity of clinical expertise. Sometimes you simply need someone who is detail-oriented, organized and familiar with the protocol involved as it relates to your issue, if it is non-medical.

To determine if a particular advocate is right for you, interview candidates carefully to make sure the advocate you choose has the right expertise and history of "wins" in similar situations. Personality, availability and business model of advocates vary widely and there should be a strong sense of correct fit with the advocate hired. The three national professional organizations— APHA, NAHAC and PPAI—have resources on their websites to help people find an advocate in their area, as well as guide them through the interview process. Just as every patient or client is unique, so are advocates.

To determine if you need an advocate, read as much as possible and listen to your gut instincts. Don't be afraid to ask for referrals and do your due diligence to become informed about this new and growing field. The field is expanding quickly, along with the growing needs of our society. In a perfect world, no one *should* need their own advocate. However, the changes occurring in the current healthcare system mean that most nurses and doctors will tell you that they don't have the time to spend with patients as much as they'd like to or as much as they used to. Everyone needs their own advocate today, whether it be a family member, a friend, or a professional.

Patient advocates fill gaps that need to be filled — to make certain the patient remains number one at all times. Patient advocates are part of the village we all need to raise a child; to save, maintain and improve the quality of a life. Readers, help us pass the word: patient advocates are here to stay because modern healthcare is complex, fast-paced, and even dangerous at times.

So: how did this epiphany come about? How did I go from being a dedicated ICU nurse for over 30 years to taking this leap of faith to become an advocate for the sick, the disabled and my favorite group, the seniors?

To begin our journey, I will share my definition of modern healthcare as it relates to our current world, as well as a couple of stories that compelled me to take action — action that changed the trajectory of my career, my life, and (I hope) the lives of those who need a village of protection to ensure their health and safety. It is my story, but many of you will find parts of yourself in it!

By the time you finish this first chapter, you'll already have a true sense of what it means to advocate for someone. You will also see, through the experiences I share, how challenging situations can escalate beyond saving, and unfortunately how, all too often, if only there were an advocate present for the patient, the outcome would not have been damaging or fatal.

You will also find "Tips to Equip" at the end of each chapter. These tips are pulled directly from sections within the chapter to equip you with information that can help you advocate for your loved ones — or on your own behalf, depending on the situation. These tips are also to educate you, so you have a better sense of what feels right and what does not; and to help you as you decide whether a patient advocate is the right fit to help you move through a challenging period of your quest for the best healthcare.

So now, let the story begin — with a few observations about values.

Over the years, I've seen a lot of people die. I have worked in ICU and oncology units in some of the best hospitals in the country over the past thirty-something years. And guess what: no one ever wishes they had worked harder or made more money on their deathbed.

Though it is true that many people want to know that their families are well provided-for, wealth is not as important as you think it might be when you are dying. The only thing that matters is whom you love and who loves you. Relationships matter.

If you hold material possessions side-by-side with your investments of love and support for your family, family wins every time. Period. We get one chance to make a difference in the world, and family is a pretty good return on investment for the vast majority of people I know. I've learned this by watching hundreds of people die over the years. It makes me more intentional about the legacy I am passing on to my own children. I hope they remember me as a person who placed people, and particularly family, far above money. Always. Even when we do not realize it, our families watch every decision we make, and I pray that I pass that value along.

I was excited about going on my first cruise to Belize at the age of 53. I had heard from my friends that a cruise was the best way to relax on vacation. To celebrate their 50th wedding anniversary, my in-laws (Nanny and Papa) decided to take their entire family on a cruise. They had realized that they had all the stuff they needed; their gift to themselves would be some uninterrupted quality time with all of their children, their spouses, and grandchildren! To me, it was a dream come true—a seven-day excursion to the Caribbean with unlimited food, endless entertainment, sun, and poolside lounge chairs where I could kick back with my entire family. An entire week's reprieve from my career as an ICU nurse! Freedom from house cleaning and all the other day-to-day duties! The grandchildren could take advantage of dozens of options for a good time while the rest of us could lounge around the pool, sipping margaritas, reading long-neglected books and taking naps whenever we felt like it. What fun we would have, all fourteen of us vacationing together! But my dream vacation turned into a medical crisis, and a patient advocate was born.

So, what happened in Belize that changed the course of our family's history and my own professional life forever?

We had a catastrophic medical emergency while we were on that cruise ship, docked off the shore of Belize. My father-in-law developed a blood clot the approximate size of Rhode Island in his inferior vena cava, the largest vein in the human body. The blood clot was lodged between his heart and his ankles, stopping blood flow to his organs, threatening to kill him at any moment. He should have gone from his stateroom directly to an intensive care unit, but there was no ICU on board that cruise ship, and no ICU where we were docked in Belize, either. Good thing he had the next best thing on board: an ICU nurse in the family. A fortunate coincidence indeed.

Looking back, I can see that we should have paid closer attention when leaving for the airport two days earlier. Papa had complained of some minor low back and hip pain, which he attributed to falling asleep in an awkward position while we were getting into the limo. We had always viewed Papa as a pretty healthy 76-year-old man, though I knew he had a hereditary disorder, called prothrombin gene mutation, that causes his blood to clot too easily. A couple of months earlier, he had experienced a fainting spell and was found to have a couple of blood clots in his lungs. Blood clots in the lungs, known as pulmonary emboli, generally begin in the legs and dislodge and travel northbound via the inferior vena cava and become lodged in the pulmonary artery, where they are often fatal dependent upon their size. Before our cruise, surgeons had placed a special filter in his vena cava (the same vein that developed the huge clot on the cruise) to prevent blood clots in his legs from reaching his lungs. This IVC (inferior vena cava) filter made us feel confident that he would not develop any serious blood clots to his lungs. Problem solved, right?

So, when Papa fainted outside the dining room two days into our cruise, we all thought it was odd, but we were not alarmed. After all, he had the filter! We were confident that it was not a blood clot. We had him checked out by the ship's doctor (a lovely South African gentleman whom I will never forget) and the plan was to have him come back for another clinic visit the next morning to make certain all was well, just to be on the safe side. We were satisfied and appreciative of the physician's concern and thorough examination.

The next morning when I arrived at Nanny and Papa's stateroom to accompany him back to the ship's medical clinic, I got quite a shock. Lying in bed was my beloved father-in-law, cold and clammy, with both legs swollen and starting to turn a nasty shade of blue (what we in the medical world call cyanosis, caused by lack of oxygen flow). Nanny said, "He's having a hard time getting to the bathroom."

I think my initial thought was, *"Holy Mother of God, we are in deep trouble now."*

Not wanting to cause undue alarm in a situation I knew was serious, I calmly asked a few questions and wanted to get Papa settled into a wheelchair so we could take him to see the ship's physician as quickly as possible. Nanny knew something wasn't right, but she did not know how sick he was. I was not about to tell her right then and risk whipping her up into hysteria. Then I would have two problems to deal with… not to mention the rest of the family!

While I was getting Papa into the wheelchair, I noticed things that others would only glance at; I was calm, confident, and hyper-alert. I realized that my father-in-law had just clotted off his IVC filter, effectively halting blood flow to his lungs from his body below the diaphragm. Body organs need blood flow. This was serious. The lack of blood flow from his legs to his upper body impeded his circulation and caused his legs to swell. The cold, clammy skin told me he was going into shock. I knew that low blood flow to his kidneys and bowel could cause serious complications if we did not restore it quickly. I noticed all of this and thought about the ramifications of it all, calmly wheeling him down the hallway to the ship's physician. I formulated in my mind what medical professionals would call a differential diagnosis and plan of care, based on my findings. I hoped I was wrong.

I watched the ship's doctor examine Papa and my alarm grew as I noticed that he wore the same calm, professional, eerily quiet demeanor that I did. I asked him out into the hall and discussed my suspicions.

"I think he's clotted off his IVC filter. What do you think?" I ventured.

The doctor nodded, relieved that I understood what was happening. "I think we have a serious problem."

Unfortunately, there was no ultrasound machine on the ship. The closest ultrasound machine was at a community hospital in Belize. Being a less-developed country, we knew it would not be a major university hospital—but we decided to take him off the ship and transfer him. They could do a diagnostic workup and we could proceed from there. At least, I reasoned, they would surely have intravenous blood thinners (like Heparin) that would prevent the clot from progressing and hopefully Papa's own body would slowly be able to break down the clot that was growing by the minute. Having been in developing countries' medical centers many times before, I was curious about what we would find in Belize. I wondered if this hospital would be able to handle a full-blown medical emergency if, God forbid, Papa's heart or lungs would stop working.

While all of this went on in my mind's eye, Papa was laughing and joking, charming the ship's nurse and medical technician, oblivious to what was about to happen. After I conveyed my suspicions to the family, they all decided that I would be the logical choice to go with him as he left the ship that day, and we all agreed to stay in close contact by cell phone. Nanny started to cry as she kissed him good-bye while everyone else stood around reassuring themselves that it would all be fine and we would reunite in a day or two. (As for me, I wasn't so sure, but I stayed calm and quiet. There was no sense in taking the entire family off the ship, as there was nothing any of them could do, and truthfully, paying attention to everyone's opinions would only distract me from the work involved in keeping a close eye on Papa. As we left the ship that day I prayed hard while staying calm and reassuring, but I was also hyper-alert for every detail, every symptom, that could herald the onset of an acute medical emergency.

We got to the hospital in Belize that day and the very tiny emergency room looked to be a slight improvement over some of the African hospitals I'd seen before, so I felt confident that they would be able to help. Treatment of choice would likely initially be Heparin through an IV to prevent further blood clots from forming, and to wait seven to 10 days for the body's normal clot/ fibrin breakdown process to dissolve the blood clot. If this had been a major medical center, Papa would have been rushed to the interventional radiology lab and had the clot manually extracted by a specially trained physician; we did not have that option in Belize. We had no way of knowing how extensive the blood clot was. An antiquated ultrasound machine was able to determine that Papa had blood clots in both of his legs, but it malfunctioned and broke down halfway through the test. The doctor's (a great man, I'll refer to here as "Dr. O") best guess was that the clots were fairly extensive, so we decided that we would admit Papa to the hospital and stay on a Heparin drip for a few days and see what happened.

For three days we stayed in the small hospital room together — I in one bed, Papa in another. He remained on bed rest with a continual infusion of Heparin to prevent further clot formation. Heparin does not actually dissolve clots; a stronger category of medicine known as thrombolytics will dissolve clots, but they are high-risk medications only given under very limited circumstances. Papa would not have qualified for those anyway due to previous medical problems related to his hereditary blood-clotting disorder. This was not an ideal treatment, but it was the best we had. We were still sitting on a ticking time bomb, hoping for the best.

The third day in the hospital was Thanksgiving. The kind hospital chef who cooked, served, and cleared the food for every patient in the facility tried hard to make our day pleasant. She did her best with a Belizean version of a Thanksgiving dinner. She was sweet and the dinner was lovely, though we missed our family very much. Everyone at the hospital was very nice: the doctor, nurses, cleaning staff, and the chef who brought us that special meal. We were grateful for all of them on that Thanksgiving Day. Little did I realize that it was the calm before the storm, and I was about to have my nursing instincts and every skill I'd learned during the course of my career tested to the very limits of my capacity.

Dr. O came into the room with some special news that day which he was certain would please us: Papa would now be allowed to get out of bed and walk to the bathroom. Papa was delighted; me, not so much. Small warning bells went off in my head and I questioned him (very politely, of course; it's always a good idea to be respectful and polite to one's healthcare providers).

"Are you sure?" I asked the doctor.

He assured me that Papa was fine and it was time to progressively increase his activity in anticipation of a quick discharge. He related his concern that older people who stay in bed too long get weaker and weaker, which I knew to be true from experience.

I went along with the plan after he left and helped Papa walk to the bathroom. Besides feeling a little dizzy, he was walking well and he looked forward to some alone time in the bathroom, away from the watchful eyes of his daughter-in-law.

As I stood outside the bathroom door that day, I struggled with two conflicting priorities. First, I wanted to guard my father-in-law's health and safety, but regretfully I also wanted to be seen by the medical staff as a source of help rather than a hindrance to his care. Nurses and doctors are used to seeing family members behaving badly in a healthcare crisis, and I did not want to be seen as a problem family member that they needed to tiptoe around. I'm a good nurse, but also a nice person, so I did not want to offend the doctor. I went along with his plan even though it made me uneasy. I knew the clot had not dissolved yet, from my knowledge of the pathophysiology of the hematological system (blood disorders, such as anemia, leukemia, and clotting disorders).

After three minutes in the bathroom, I called out to Papa: "Are you okay in there?"

I got no answer.

I knocked on the door and heard him mumble, "I don't feel so good…"

I opened the door and my jaw dropped. Standing before me was my father-in-law, quickly turning the darkest shade of purple I had ever seen anyone turn and still be alive. He was dying right before my eyes. So, I quickly did what any seasoned ICU nurse would do: I put my emotions up on a shelf and initiated the emergency response system, calling a code blue.

As I called for help and half-carried Papa back to bed, lifting his feet up higher than his head onto pillows, I soon breathed a sigh of relief as the blood started returning to his face and he became more alert. It took us several minutes to read even a blood pressure of 50/30. The blood flow to his brain and heart had been severely impaired due to the extensive clot that acted as a beaver's dam in his vena cava, the main river of the circulatory system. Everything downstream of his clotted-off IVC filter was backing up, and his body could not break down the clot quickly enough. I saw that he could not stand up for more than a minute or two without becoming symptomatic, so I knew the clot was going to need more aggressive intervention than the Heparin drip he had been receiving. All this I knew from my past clinical experience and finely-honed assessment skills from decades of ICU bedside nursing. Book knowledge is one thing, but clinical savvy is worth its weight in gold when dealing with acute medical emergencies. Doctors and nurses have told me for years how glad they are when I am running the code in hospitals. They value clinical experience, as well, and they know how important it is to stay calm and collected as you multi-task in the midst of a CODE situation.

It was, however, a completely new challenge to try to save the life of a family member. Our beloved patriarch's life was literally in my hands now, and it scared me nearly to my own death. After making certain he was stabilizing, I excused myself to the bathroom for a few minutes and had a good cry before launching into the next leg of our journey. I came out of the bathroom with firm resolve to move quickly so that I could get him back to the U.S.; he could get appropriate emergency treatment there.

The entire medical and nursing staff gathered around Papa's bed in the Belizean hospital that day, the doctor looking sheepishly down at his shoes, a nervous tic around his left temple. I took a deep breath after seeing Papa's blood pressure slowly return to normal; he became more alert and wondered what had just happened. I turned to the doctor, who minutes earlier had assured me that his patient would be just fine to get out of bed that day, and said simply, "We're going back to the U.S. today."

The next few hours were a blur of phone calls, requesting copies of tests and X-rays and speaking with the travel insurance carrier that my in-laws had wisely contracted prior to the trip. It would take too long to get a special MED-EVAC plane into this tiny Caribbean community, so we compromised for the sake of expediency. The first plane leaving for Miami would depart in three hours, so the agent booked two first-class seats and I instructed the attendants that he would not be allowed to stand up for any reason. He would fly with his head reclined and feet up all the way back home to Chicago, going through customs in Miami with an escort and an ICU nurse at his side. He was carried up the steps to the plane in a wheelchair.

The trip back to Chicago was stressful for me, but hey—I'm an ICU nurse and I thrive on excitement. Put me in a classroom with twenty-five children for an hour and I will have a nervous breakdown, but put me in an ICU with the sickest patient they have, and I am in my element. I love helping to save people's lives for a living. Holistic nursing—providing physical, emotional, and spiritual support to people in great need, is what I do best. It is extremely rewarding and has made me a better human being. I am proud to be a nurse. It's one of the most nobel professions there is, despite how much harder it has gotten in recent years.

As I sat next to Papa that day on the plane and stayed by his side as we made our way back to the U.S., I played my role well—alert but not alarmist. I knew deep down that Papa could die at any moment; the change in cabin pressure could trigger a sudden catastrophic event, but we had no choice but to try to get home, closer to the high-tech equipment that could save him.

People who are not physically healthy should not fly. If they are *really* unhealthy, they may not even be stable enough to travel several hours home by ambulance. I've had patients who begged to go home on hospice when their cancer grew worse in spite of treatment, and they died on the way home. That's tough for families to live with.

Once we arrived at O'Hare and settled into a limousine headed for our community's largest hospital, we were both breathing a little easier. Finally, our ordeal would be over soon. Our safe haven was in sight.

We arrived at the hospital ER at about 1:00 a.m. and explained to the triage nurse at the front desk that Papa was in the midst of a medical emergency. Unfortunately, dear Papa became a charming businessman again, which works well—when negotiating business deals. He turned on the charm and chatted amiably with the ER nurse, looking for all the world as if he were still on vacation. As he sat in the wheelchair with no complaints whatsoever, he really did not look sick. The triage nurse probably relayed that impression to the physician as well. After a few minutes of pleasant conversation, we were ushered into an ER bay and I helped him get onto the cart and put on a hospital gown. A few moments passed and a new doctor, Dr. C, walked in. We relayed the events of the past four days and he listened politely, making a few notes on Papa's paper chart. After a few more questions and polite nods of the head, the doctor excused himself to call my father-in-law's primary care physician. I was certain that Papa would soon be admitted and scheduled for an early interventional radiology procedure the next morning.

Now, to be fair to the ER doctor, I never tell people I am an ICU nurse when I show up with family members to the ER. I want to see how common folk are treated. I think everyone should be treated equally in a hospital, and I don't want anyone assuming anything about me either just because I'm a nurse. My feeling is that if a hospital treats all patients with respect, kindness, and highly competent care in an ER, then the hospital probably has a culture of premium quality care.

So, when Dr. C came back to deliver his diagnosis and plan of care, I was all ears.

He said, "I called Dr. M and told him what's going on with you, and Dr. M said that these things happen sometimes, and you can go home on subcutaneous Lovenox (a form of blood thinner less potent than the Heparin drip he had been on in Belize) and you should be fine."

You can imagine the long silence from me.

After collecting myself for a few seconds, I could hold it in no longer. I crossed my arms, looked into the doctor's eyes, and said firmly, "We just told you all the reasons why I believe my father-in-law has clotted off his IVC filter. He cannot even stand up without passing out. He has a blood clot that is turning into concrete from his diaphragm all the way down both legs. Look at his feet! We are not going anywhere until he goes to the interventional lab and they inject dye into his vena cava that proves me wrong. You go call Dr. T [my cardiologist friend] and tell him that Teri Dreher is in the ER with her father-in-law and she is being difficult. He'll know what to do. We are not going anywhere, sir."

The good doctor had probably started to realize by now that I was in the medical field. He politely excused himself to call Dr. T. Within three minutes, he returned and shared that Dr. T wanted my father-in-law admitted and scheduled for a venogram at 8:00 a.m.

Papa had never seen me get riled up before, so in the days to come, he relayed to all his friends how Teri had assertively interacted with the ER physician. Ever since then, whenever the story comes up, I always tell my family to remember that nice doctors are not always right. Just because they stride confidently into your room and tell you what *should* happen does not mean you need to go along with their plan. It's a joint decision. ER doctors have about five minutes to spend with each patient and thirty minutes to spend with their chart. They don't have time to hear every minute detail of your past medical history. Be polite, be respectful of their time, but remember that you know your family member better than anyone, so trust your instincts and question the plan if it doesn't feel right.

The next morning when I arrived at 7:30 a.m., Papa was already in the interventional radiology lab. An interventional radiology lab is like a heart catheterization lab (where heart attacks are treated). They are run by interventional radiologists—physicians who are experts at reading x-rays, CT scans, and MRIs, but have also had extensive training in a wide variety of minimally invasive vascular procedures that save people's lives every day. Think of an interventional radiologist as a cream-of-the-crop radiologist with a surgeon's personality. They are the gods of the radiology world! The physician emerged from the room four and a half hours later, telling us he had never seen such an extensive clot. He used a microscopic high-tech drill and employed multiple attempts to free the clot and open his circulation once more, restoring blood flow to his legs and vital organs. What a relief!

After his procedure in the interventional radiology lab, Papa went to the ICU that day for recovery and, once again, we optimistically assumed that he would quickly recover and we would all be on our way out the door soon.

It was not to be.

My dear father-in-law endured every complication known to man, and our family witnessed firsthand the best and worst of medical care over the ensuing two months. After the first few near-death experiences, my friend Dr. T contacted a colleague at Rush Presbyterian St. Luke's Hospital in Chicago who happened to be one of the world's top experts in rare congenital clotting disorders. These doctors, Dr. T and Dr. V, saved my father-in-law's life. Rush's team of expert interventional radiologists performed multiple life-saving procedures; Dr. L did a procedure on him that stopped persistent bleeding, though it had only been done experimentally twice before. I am grateful for these doctors.

They are heroes and our family will be forever grateful to every one of them.

During the six weeks of Papa's hospitalizations in Belize and Illinois, I had a chance to view the hospital experience from the inside out, as a family member. This completely foreign vantage point was, for me, a very valuable learning experience — an epiphany of sorts. Communication problems between practitioners, multiple crises requiring emergent surgical procedures, allergic reactions to medicines, almost bleeding to death, descending into hemorrhagic shock, and several ICU admissions convinced me of the great need for professional advocacy.

What would have happened if I had not been with our beloved patriarch when disaster struck? The entire family affirmed that they knew he would have died if I had not been there. I was just doing my job and thinking of little else but standing guard, watching and observing, asking all the right questions, and asserting myself if I felt he was not receiving the best care. I knew my father-in-law better than any of the care providers did, plus I had the advantage of advanced clinical expertise. Not many families have that luxury. Fortunately, my father-in-law is healthier today than he was in 2008 and we had a positive outcome. Sadly, not everyone is so fortunate.

When I returned to work after our family's six-week ordeal, I had new eyes and new empathy to truly understand what families go through, and I began to advocate even more strongly for patient safety. A few months later, I came close to being fired over advocating for a patient who was having multiple complications from a major surgery. When I asked the surgeon why my patient was not being sent for scans and exploratory surgery for multiple episodes of bleeding, I soon found myself on a ten-day suspension from work for a charting omission. During a CODE on that same patient, I neglected to scan out a narcotic properly — and the hospital essentially accused me of being a drug abuser and escorted me to the door while we waited for the drug screen results.

To clarify, I'm sure my suspension had nothing to do with the charting omission error; those omissions happen all the time. Though I was still satisfied in my heart that I had made the right decision to stand up for the patient and question the surgeon's judgment, I heard the message loud and clear: nurses who stand up against powerful, money-making surgeons, and threaten the image of the hospital by drawing attention to errors, can quickly find themselves labeled "expendable." Nurses have a bill of rights just as patients do, and one of our rights states that we should not be persecuted for advocating for patients, but the facts can be twisted any way facilities want them to — and who wants to fight big business?

Many nurses are playing it safe these days, keeping their heads down and not making waves unless they have to. We are the ambassadors for the hospitals and we are to provide quality care, avoid errors, and make the hospital look good. This is a tall order, considering the time constraints that our computers demand. Nursing takes a toll on our minds, hearts, and backs. A looming shortage of nurses and primary care physicians is predicted to peak in 2018. It will be interesting to watch how the hospital industry endeavors to fill the gaps — as well as how the shortages will affect patient care. Something's gotta give.

What is modern healthcare?

I tread lightly here as I share some of my impressions of what modern healthcare means to me as a career nurse. I have seen it from the inside and the outside, and I know what you are going through if you have had frustrations with modern healthcare. I have seen the fear, outrage, and shock as our family went through our own medical calamity, and I know it is not an isolated incident. I've also seen modern healthcare (in its current incarnation) from years of studying the Affordable Care Act. From my point of view, modern healthcare falls under two very large umbrellas: the quality of healthcare and the financial ramifications stemming from the inception of the Affordable Care Act.

There are no villains in the world of modern healthcare, but the U.S. system is fractured and it's not always safe going into the hospital for a multitude of reasons. I think it's safe to say it will be a long while before America has her healthcare mess straightened out; in its prior state, the system was not sustainable with costs running away as they were before Barack Obama signed the ACA into law.

From a financial standpoint, however, there is little affordable about the Affordable Care Act. Healthcare costs are still rising, albeit at a somewhat slower pace. The costs of insurance have risen at least 40 percent for those paying for private insurance, and deductibles have never been higher. Out-of-pocket medical expenses are higher than ever as well. Insurance brokers are going out of business at record rates since commissions have been cut down or eliminated, and the insurance landscape is changing daily.

The Affordable Care Act, or "Obamacare" as it is often called, is the most radical change within the system to which modern healthcare refers. Whether you are a liberal or conservative, there are many vantage points that are valid when looking at the ACA from different perspectives. There are many wonderful provisions of the ACA: closing of the donut hole for Medicare recipients, making drug costs more affordable, free prevention screenings for cancer, yearly free physicals (as long as no treatment or problems are addressed), ambulatory services, emergency care, maternity and mental health services, etc. The benefits to the Medicaid population cannot be overstated; and general access to healthcare for the poor has improved, especially in urban areas. Detractors still say that it places undue restrictions on physicians to deliver care they know their patients need. Doctors can no longer just think about the patient; they must think about insurance limitations, costs, ICD-10 codes (used to code the patient's diagnosis for insurance companies to pay claims for services rendered) and charting correctly, which takes time. Rarely do physicians and nurses have time to read a patient's whole chart, so important details are missed all the time.

According to the *Examiner*, New Jersey family physician Dr. John Tedeschi said, "Just as a guitar string must be tuned, so does a person's health to get the right tone. The government has taken away, or refocused the intelligence part of the tuning, and has just about destroyed the creative, or compassion component. Now under Obamacare, we are left with an incompetent mechanism that does not have the best interests of the patient in mind."

Another physician friend of mine, Dr. T, describes deep discouragement at working so hard to build up a successful cardiology practice, only to have to spend over $25,000 on new computers that would comply with government regulations for electronic health record charting. At the same time, his practice had to stop doing stress tests in the office with the new equipment they had just bought—because reimbursement rates favored hospital-based stress tests after Obamacare was enacted. Many doctors are struggling to keep their practice focused on patient care, but due to the sheer amount of documentation required for insurance accounting purposes, doctors feel that their attention is diverted away from patient care in favor of computer work. Many approach retirement discouraged and worried about how their aging patients will fare in this new healthcare landscape.

Not all doctors are so negative towards post-ACA medicine. In large part, doctors are split along political party lines, with 87 percent of physicians who lean towards the Democratic Party reporting that they feel "mostly positive" about the impact of Obamacare. In contrast, the exact same number of Republicans felt it had a negative impact on quality, safety and cost. Independents tended to lean toward a more negative opinion, according to a study published by Kaiser Health in 2015.

Though many will agree that the ACA has had a negative financial impact on patients, if questioned, they realize that the state of American healthcare could not continue without drastic change. The U.S. has the most expensive healthcare system in the world and it is far from the highest quality. In fact, the World Health Organization rates U.S. healthcare somewhere between #25 and #27 in terms of quality, safety and cost. A study published by the Wall Street Journal in June of 2016 showed that medical error is *still* the third leading cause of death in America today. Why is it so dangerous to be a patient in hospitals today in America?

A comprehensive overview can be found in a landmark study from 1999: "To Err is Human: Building a Better Healthcare System." The study claimed that about 30 percent of patients who enter a hospital will incur some sort of "adverse medical outcome," which is code for medical error. It can be something as simple as an allergic reaction to a new medication — or something as extreme as a wrong body part being removed, or sponges left inside the body during surgery that leads to sepsis (a blood infection) and even death.

The quality of healthcare has declined, the numbers of medical errors are on the rise, and excellent physicians and nurses are leaving their professions in large numbers. This does not bode well for healthcare in the United States.

The statistics are there to back up what we have observed: many physicians have left private practice or are thinking of leaving medicine due to the heavy demands placed upon them (Jauhar, 2014). Physicians are disheartened with medicine. In a survey of 12,000 physicians, only six percent said their morale was positive. The truth is: we all need physicians, and we don't want to see them leaving their profession.

So, why are physicians leaving practice? In a Wall Street Journal article entitled "Why Doctors are Sick of Their Profession" (Jauhar, 2014), Dr. Sandeep Jauhar reminisces how physicians in the mid-twentieth century were "the pillars of any community," and how becoming a physician was a noble profession. Doctors were free to set their own hours and their own fees, and they practiced medicine without answering to administrative restrictions. As medicine began to become more highly managed with the development of HMOs in the 1970's, physicians' decision-making autonomy decreased, as did physician compensation. This has only worsened with the ACA: reimbursement has decreased further and administrative entanglements keep doctors from seeing patients as often as they'd like. Still, due to the individual mandate in the ACA, doctors did see an uptick in patients, even if they couldn't spend as much time with patients as they may have liked. Under the Trump administration's new tax law, states will have more control over ACA requirements. Depending on state party lines, physicians may see some major changes coming their way, specifically with the rollback of the individual mandate.

Today's physicians are financially struggling. Many people assume that doctors are all rich; these days, physician income is lower due to increased expenses in operating a medical practice (particularly malpractice insurance premiums) and lower reimbursement rates from insurance companies. Again, this could be changing soon, but as of 2017, studies cite that physicians are now making less money per year than 20 years ago while seeing twice as many patients per day.

With medical malpractice suits at an all-time high, physicians are paying exorbitant premiums for their malpractice insurance. One fine doctor had such a high malpractice insurance premium that he remarked, "The day that my malpractice exceeds my income, I'm outta here!" Sadly, many excellent physicians share his sentiments.

Then there's the issue of low reimbursement rates by private insurance carriers and Medicare. A physician may bill, for example, $1800 for performing a colonoscopy, and only be paid $200 by the patient's insurance company. The low reimbursement puts physicians under pressure to work faster and see more patients in a day to make ends meet. Add in the fact that student loan debt has become a bigger and bigger issue for medical students and the stress of high performance is even more prevalent.

To increase the number of patients seen in a day (and thus increase office revenue), some doctors have resorted to hiring physician assistants (PA's); this is not ideal either as it brings the other component of the modern healthcare umbrella into play: quality care. It might surprise you how little training a PA has compared to a physician. Your physician must first earn an undergraduate degree, then attend four years of medical school (two years spent "in the books" and two years spent in the hospitals experiencing hands-on learning). After those four years, they may then be called Doctor. Physicians then spend a year in an internship and during that year, they apply for a residency position. Residency can last anywhere from three to seven years depending upon the medical specialty they have chosen.

In contrast, a PA's training consists of completing an undergraduate college degree and then only two years obtaining a master's degree in Physician Assistant Practice before they are off examining, diagnosing, and treating patients. How can this be? PAs are physician assistants, but the physician who employs the PA is liable for their work as well as their own.

It used to be that the physician had to be present in the office while the PA was seeing patients, and their charts had to be countersigned by the physician, but that has changed too. Over 29 states have passed legislation that allows PAs to see patients without countersignature by a physician (Japsen, 2016).

In this era of everyone suing one another, physicians live with a constant worry of being sued, of missing something, yet their hands are tied by insurance company policies that require pre-approval (which sometimes result in non-approval of coverage) for important tests like CT scans, MRIs and the like. Want to have some blood work done? The physician had better come up with legitimate diagnoses that justify the tests, or they won't be paid for. This certainly contributes to low morale.

While electronic medical records were devised to help hospitals ensure accuracy and efficiency, they put newfound stress on almost all hospital staff. EMRS are a constant thorn in physicians' sides. Where once the patient was the focus of care and doctors could spend the time necessary to listen to their patients, thoroughly examine them, and carefully think through treatment plans, now the computer takes center stage. One doctor described the hospital's "documentation specialists," hospital employees whose job it is to make sure that all documentation will yield the best payment from the insurance company, as a constant source of harassment to doctors. He spoke of floods of emails reminding him of some omission in the unwieldy computer charting system. These types of emails are unpleasant distractions and aggravations in the lives of talented and caring physicians; they'd rather focus on the patients than on the computer! Hospitals' medical record departments routinely send doctors threatening letters telling them that their hospital privileges will be removed if they do not get caught up with their charting, and it's getting harder and harder to get caught up these days.

It's no wonder that many excellent primary care physicians are giving in to the pressure to allow physicians known as hospitalists to manage their patients when they go into the hospital. A hospitalist is a physician, usually an internal medicine specialist, employed by the hospital to care for inpatients. That means the patient's private physician won't even come and see them while they're in the hospital. Most patients, especially seniors, would much rather have their personal physician manage their care when they are hospitalized. One woman mentioned that she saw three different hospitalists and two specialists when she was in the hospital. She had no idea who was handling what! This isn't just an inconvenience for patients who want to see someone they know. Primary care physicians are one of the top ways to keep people healthy and out of the hospital. Utilizing and maintaining a relationship with a primary care physician yields better health outcomes across the board.

Our broken system and burned-out physicians are compromising what used to be excellent care. Physicians used to be willing to take care of patients without financial resources because it was the right thing to do. Today, they are stretched so far that most practices cannot do this anymore. Many are refusing Medicaid and even Medicare patients, due to lower reimbursement rates.

There is a shortage of primary care physicians, and it's expected to get much worse. Many primary care physicians have now reached retirement age, and primary care is not an area that many new graduates want to get into because of low reimbursement, long hours, and high student loan debt. Having fewer primary care physicians hurts everyone. According to a CBS news report, "[The] future shortage is especially troubling due to the growing needs patients are expected to have as the American population continues to age" (cbsnews.com).

Registered nurses are leaving their profession as well. When I started my health consultancy business, North Shore Patient Advocates (now NShore Patient Advocates), in the fall of 2011, it was largely a result of my father-in-law's health crisis in the hospitals in Belize and Illinois. I saw the cracks in our increasingly complex healthcare system from a family member's perspective. At the time, I was an ICU nurse with 38 years of strong clinical experience. I had also worked as a cardiovascular nurse clinician for a busy interventional cardiologist. I was comfortable with handling complex medical and surgical patients with multi-system pathology. I loved the pace of the intensive care unit and had always been a natural patient advocate. I spoke up for patients and families, and offered physical, emotional, and spiritual support to those in crisis. And I still loved the art and practice of bedside nursing, but I had never experienced firsthand the terror and frustration that families experience when a loved one has a medical crisis.

But nursing has changed from how I was trained in school, and from how I practiced for most of my career. As one of their many excellent qualities, nurses are taught to utilize keen powers of observation and to critically analyze tests and clinical findings.

Sadly, the time that we used to spend doing that is now being severely reduced by excessive computerized medical record-keeping requirements needed to protect the hospital's liability. The new mantra is, "If it didn't get charted, it didn't happen." Whereas it used to take 20-30 minutes per day to chart by hand, we now have to spend two to three hours per patient per day feeding the computer monster. I cannot count how many times I have spent over an hour charting a morning assessment, only to run to attend to an emergent patient need without saving my data and poof! All of that data is gone, and I must start the entire process over again.

Nurses now attend seminars solely dedicated to "how to cover our butts above all else." This is frustrating for caring individuals with a passion to help and heal. We don't want to spend all our time tending to computers. Most personal care in hospitals is now provided by certified nursing assistants (CNAs). CNAs complete a certificate program, typically three months in length at a junior college, so naturally they don't have the same powers of observation and critical thinking as registered nurses. We are eternally grateful for their help, however. Nurses are drowning in technology and we all miss our patients; CNAs are to nurses what nurse practitioners and physician assistants are to doctors. We all need help doing our jobs.

In his Wall Street Journal article, Dr. Jauhar made an astute statement: "Unhappy doctors make for unhappy patients." He remarked, "For many of us, it is rare to find a primary physician who can remember us from visit to visit, let alone come to know us in depth or with any meaning or relevancy."

Not long ago, a woman came to us with a plea to help her son. He had previously been admitted to a hospital with a kidney stone that was causing severe pain. The urologist had placed a stent into the man's kidney and bladder to allow the stone to pass. Since the stent was so uncomfortable, the young man had been unable to return to his job as a laborer. And since he had no insurance, he applied for Medicaid at the hospital, but was told it would be several weeks or months before he would be approved.

When it was time to have the stent removed, the young man called the surgeon's office to set up the appointment for the removal but was told that unless he could come up with $1,000 cash, he would not be seen and the stent would not be removed. The patient had submitted proof that he was doing all that he could to get covered by Medicaid. Unfortunately, Medicaid now reimburses physicians at such low rates that many practitioners refuse to accept Medicaid patients.

41

The paradox: this unfortunate young man, unable to work due to the pain from the stent, yet unable to have it removed without cash in hand, would have been forced to go to an emergency room and accrue another large hospital bill for pain control and to force someone's hand to remove the stent. These are some of the harsh realities facing modern healthcare: people are still falling through the cracks. We see it every day.

My heart broke for this young man. Even though he could not afford a private advocate, we decided to take his case on a pro-bono basis. It was unethical to allow this patient to stay in pain simply because he had no money.

Fortunately, this story has a happy ending: when we intervened as this young man's private patient advocate, the surgeon's office was very accommodating in scheduling the stent removal. The patient was happy to have his story shared in hopes of educating and inspiring others. As healthcare professionals, we all take an oath to follow a code of ethics, and there are times and circumstances where it would be unethical to refuse service for financial reasons.

The new healthcare landscape (which is constantly evolving, still) is about money, marketing, statistics, and efficiency. We are in quite a pickle; my concern for patients today is for their safety. Modern healthcare is splitting into fragments, and the patient must remain at the center of the model of care.

While it is almost impossible for healthcare professionals to keep up with the changes, there are signs of hope on the horizon. I remain confident that we will eventually settle into a fair and reasonable place. Grassroots efforts, such as the exploding field of professional advocacy, are one of the many possible solutions on the horizon.

Chapter 2

Private Professional Healthcare Advocates: Another Level

Darla's story is an important part of why I left a successful career as an ICU nurse. She made me see modern healthcare in a whole new light; after my experience during her crises, I realized how far healthcare has drifted. I will never forget her story.

Without a doubt, the following account brought the stark reality of marketing, money and the hierarchy of power in large corporations to the forefront, for me. I quickly learned the career dangers attached to making decisions from too far down the food chain. It made me see how impotent we are as nurses when things go awry and we have the audacity to call attention to them.

I never know which patients I will fall in love with, but Darla and her extraordinary family were easy to love. Darla came to us when other hospitals told her to go home and get her affairs in order because her cancer was far too advanced to treat. She had a particularly aggressive form of cancer that had invaded her entire abdominal cavity. The metastasis was extensive and she came to us looking for hope. She underwent an aggressive surgical procedure that required her to be in ICU for several weeks and her course of recovery was fraught with multiple complications. She came close to bleeding to death on several occasions and I began to wonder why her episodes of hemorrhage were not investigated more carefully by her surgical team.

One day I approached her surgeon and asked why he had not sent her for studies to determine the origin of her bleeding. I asked him, "Help me understand where you think the bleeding is coming from."

To say my inquiries were not well received is an understatement. Without answers for his failure to investigate the cause of her hemorrhaging, the surgeon's only response was to take a defensive and angry stance. He began to sputter nonsensical justifications and made it very clear that a mere nurse was not to question his authority. Within 24 hours, he had ordered my unstable patient to be transferred to the step-down unit.

He would have been better off waving a red flag in front of a bull.

I am not afraid of physicians who get angry and defensive because I have always been just idealistic enough to believe that it takes a coordinated team effort to bring healing to any patient. I was married to a physician for ten years and I know that they are human just like we are: fallible, imperfect, and doing their best to give their patients a second, third, or even fourth chance at life. It takes a special kind of boldness to be a surgeon: to cut into another human being's flesh and slice into their inner parts, sewing and repairing broken organs infected with disease. I admire that boldness and courage greatly and have the greatest respect for the hundreds of fine surgeons I have had the privilege to work with closely.

Most doctors will tell you that a good ICU nurse is a surgeon's best friend, especially in community hospitals without residents on call while many times, working twenty-four hours per day. I love working with great doctors and I love making their job easier.

It's a great team experience and the mutual respect I have always enjoyed makes being an ICU nurse more fun than anything I can ever imagine. We get to save lives and help quell people's suffering every day we go to work. Who could ask for a better profession?

On this particular day, the doctor I was talking to did not welcome my questions—or the threat that they posed to his position. I still don't understand why he did not come to the unit when she was bleeding the day I questioned him. I will never understand why he didn't try harder to get to the root of her complications earlier until he was ultimately forced to do so. Did it have anything to do with the fact that she was African-American? I hope not, but there is evidence in hospitals around the country that black patients do not receive the most aggressive treatment in comparison to white patients. Darla was a highly successful and educated woman, a banker, with devoted and educated children who stayed at her bedside for weeks. They kept careful notes and asked questions constantly.

This was a beautiful family, one that I got to know well over her weeks-long stay in the ICU. When she had several hemorrhages that caused her to vomit quarts of blood, her hair would become matted and her body would be severely weakened by the trauma involved in resuscitating her. I remember several times when I would wash her hair, bathe her and lovingly apply lotions and creams to make her feel beautiful again after such episodes. The final ritual involved putting on her makeup and inserting her special signature gold hoop earrings back in place. She was a dignified woman and it was important to help restore her dignity after her medical crises. We even celebrated her birthday in the ICU in grand style, complete with singing, laughter, and balloons.

I learned many years ago how important the little things are to patients. When my father-in-law had a crisis in Belize, it never occurred to me to take legal action against Dr.O. Mistakes happen and no permanent damage was done. What I remember most is how kind and helpful the staff was when we arrived and when we were arranging our trip back to the US. In our time of need, they were there. When nurses and clinicians take the time to show loving kindness to their patients, it speaks volumes to their worth and value; I truly believe it helps people find comfort and healing in the worst of medical crises. Care and comfort is woven into the fabric of who nurses are; it's just as important as any of the technical or assessment skills we possess. It is one of the reasons why nursing has ranked at the top of the Barna research polls for decades as the single most trusted profession by the public.

When I challenged the doctor on that day ten years ago, he was angry enough to contact hospital administrators. Next, he directed his mid-level support staff to transfer Darla to another floor the following day. Later that afternoon, Darla's daughter came up to the ICU and pleaded with me for help. "I'm afraid Mommy is going to die, Teri! Her blood pressure is 60/40 and she has been lying in bloody stools for the last half hour. The nurses don't have time to clean her up. Please help us!" I assured her that something would be done and contacted my nurse manager for help in returning her to the Intensive Care Unit.

After going downstairs and talking with the medical team, she returned and told me the doctor was not willing to bring her back to the ICU, there was nothing more she could do. My mind was racing now: I would either have to buck the system or stand by and do nothing. The director of nursing was out of town that week, so my only recourse was to go to a higher level of authority for help. I wrote an email to the hospital's CEO and asked that the risk management department become involved. Hospital risk managers are in charge of damage control when things go wrong. We needed administrative support; things were definitely going wrong.

That same day, Darla's medical situation remained unstable and her daughter came back to the ICU in tears, again asking for help. I pulled her into an empty room and said to her, "Crystal, if this was my mother, this is what I would do: I would ask the surgical team to take your mom to the interventional lab for a CAT scan to investigate the source of her bleeding, and return her to the ICU again. If they are unwilling to do that, tell them that you are going to talk to hospital administration and the risk management department. I know that my job will be in jeopardy if they find out that I told you to do this, but I don't care. We have to get your mom back to the ICU."

Things began to happen after she followed through. I was called to take Darla to the CAT scan department and to the interventional radiology department, where testing showed that she had a splenic artery aneurysm that could not be accessed by catheters needed to place a patch on the bleeding blood vessel. During the three-hour procedure, I stayed by Darla's head and prayed with her, explained what was happening, and spoke words of comfort and encouragement to her. The procedure was long and arduous, and the wonderful physicians tried everything possible to stop her bleeding. After we were done, I got her ready to transport back to the ICU and rushed her back upstairs, since her blood pressure was still dangerously low in spite of medications and blood transfusions given during the procedure.

As we wheeled her into the ICU, Darla suddenly sat up in the cart and started vomiting massive quantities of blood, with clots as big as my hand. She became cold and clammy and we rushed her into the hospital bed and called a CODE Blue. The entire medical team arrived and she was intubated, placed on life support, and the blood bank notified that we needed as much blood as they could provide for her ASAP.

The surgeon was now at the bedside, screaming orders and pacing back and forth, yelling at us to go faster as we hung blood products, poured in IV fluids, and set up vasopressors needed to save her life. For the next three and a half hours we worked feverishly to save her. We gave her over thirty units of blood products and multiple medications, including pain meds and sedation to help her stay calm during the crisis. At one point, I gave a narcotic to her in her IV and turned around to hang another unit of blood, forgetting to return later to sign out the medication with the computer scanner. That small distraction almost cost me my job.

Darla made it through that day and she stabilized in the ICU over the next week. The family requested a care conference with the entire medical team to determine the next course of action. We had the team meeting in the administration department of the hospital and the surgeon's partner arrived to explain the plan of care and answer the family's questions. He was a wise and thoughtful man and explained her condition and our options carefully, which satisfied the family. Unfortunately, Darla's aneurysm was in a unique spot that was difficult to get to non-surgically and she was not stable enough to go through another major surgical procedure. The hospital agreed to have an outside specialist consult and explore other options for treatment, but this ultimately did not resolve her challenging condition.

The family walked away from that meeting with a better understanding of her complex situation, satisfied with the answers they received that day. They thanked me for arranging for the meeting and told me later that the only reason they did not seek a medical malpractice attorney's help was because they trusted me and all that had been done to find a way to help her. Sadly, Darla died a couple of weeks later after a final massive bleeding episode. By then, the family had decided that she should not be put on life support again since her condition was not treatable. She died on my day off that week and I grieved for a war that was ultimately lost after many battles to save her life. Losing Darla broke my heart.

The following day I returned to work and before the family left the area, they came to the hospital to say goodbye to me and thank us all for working so hard to save Darla. As I embraced her daughter, she whispered in my ear that she wanted me to have a small gift to remember them by. She placed a small package in my palm. I saw that she had given me Darla's special earrings: a set of gold hoops that we had put on after every time we had cleaned her up from her bleeding episodes. They were a beautiful reminder of Darla's smile and the happy times we had spent together during her stay in the ICU. I burst into tears and thanked Crystal for this special gift, given from the heart, a reminder forever after of why patient advocacy is so important.

Today, I call these my lucky earrings and wear them every time I am asked to speak in public. This small ritual helps me remember why I do what I do. I am a professional nurse advocate and I will persevere with all my future clients to speak up on their behalf, using my experience and expertise to help them stay in the center of the model of care. It is my life's mission now.

A couple of weeks after Darla died, I was working hard to save the life of another patient with post-op bleeding. He was a lovely gentleman and I talked and laughed with him as I explained our plan for the day, hanging several units of blood. My nurse manager called me out of the room and told me she had been asked to escort me to the Occupational Health department. What for, I wondered? I was healthy and this was an inconvenient time since I was busy with my patient who needed another unit of blood.

She told me that I needed to do a urine drop exam, since I had been accused of stealing narcotics. One of the doses of pain medication had not been properly scanned out during Darla's CODE Blue weeks earlier and they had to make sure I was not stealing drugs from a patient for my own use. One of the surgeon's assistants had found my error and reported it to administration. I stood there with my jaw dropped, wondering if they had lost their mind. I had been the hospital's top ICU nurse for decades. I showed none of the classic signs of a drug-abusing nurse. I had taken the most difficult cases and the most challenging assignments for years. I was a nurse mentor, educator, and leader. Patients had sent multiple letters commending me to hospital administration. How could they think I would do something so heinous after knowing me so well for so many years? I don't know whether I was more shocked or more insulted. I know for certain that I was enraged.

As my manager escorted me to the Occupational Health department, I shook my head in disbelief. I told her over and over again that this was so wrong, so unkind, so unfair. It slowly dawned upon me that nobody *actually* thought that I was a nurse addict. The point was that I should never, ever go up against a physician who made millions of dollars a year for the hospital. Who is a hospital going to side with when a nurse blows the whistle? Nurses are, in the long run, expendable. Talented, high-profile doctors who make big money for hospitals are much harder to lose. Point taken.

In the end, this doctor actually did me a great favor. My ten-day suspension from work (why does it take ten days to get a urine screen back?) gave me a valuable opportunity to review my career direction and my options for the future. I remember telling my husband that week, in the midst of tears, anger, and hurt: "No one will ever tell me again that I cannot advocate for a patient!"

I carefully investigated patient advocacy programs around the country and signed up for one in Arizona that specifically trained experienced nurses in the business of professional advocacy. RN patient advocates equipped me to be able to start my own advocacy company. The trajectory of my career was changing, thanks to a very painful experience at that hospital. That pain was a gift in disguise.

Tips to Equip: Getting more help when you know something isn't right

1. Physicians and specialists have been trained to practice in an area of expertise that is on a higher level, so it's difficult to question their knowledge, authority, or recommendations. However, when you know that there may be more to the issue you or your loved one are experiencing, don't just settle for their word... especially if your gut is telling you differently.

2. Communication is key. The right communication is as polite and respectful as you would expect in return, but that doesn't mean you should bow down to their opinion if you feel strongly that more needs to be done. After all, they are in the *practice* of medicine; they're not perfect either.

3. When all else fails, move up the hospital food chain to achieve the results you need. Ask for a meeting with risk management and a care team conference. This lets the facility know you are an advocate for yourself or your loved one, and your concerns won't be easily dismissed simply because you don't have clinical credentials.

Next, you will become more familiar with the term "private professional healthcare advocate," or PPHA. There are various levels to patient advocacy, and this book will help you understand the difference between them all. Some will have your best interests at heart and some have their loyalties somewhere else. By the time you finish reading this section, you will see how easy it is to find the best advocate for your needs — and how it can make all the difference in the outcome of the situation you (or your loved one) may be facing. Pay close attention, because the requirements for each need are different; and you are the best one to decide which type of advocate will be the best fit for you.

Hospital advocates have a loyalty to preserve the best interests of the hospital that pays them. Their job is to ensure that risk is minimized for the hospital and its staff-particularly on the clinical side. They work for the risk management department of the hospital. Nice people — some are even nurses — but don't expect them to make leaps and bounds for you. They get their paycheck from the hospital.

Insurance company advocates are paid by the insurance company; therefore, they must look out for the best interests of the insurance company. Their job is to ensure that all of the administrative pieces are put in place to absolve the insurance company of financial responsibility, whenever possible. They have algorithms to follow, and all they know about the patient is what's on their computer screen.

For instance, if a patient receives costly medical care with an out-of-network provider, the advocate may be on the claims and/ or denials team to help decide if the treatment (any or all of it) was medically necessary. Is there any way the patient can bear some of the financial responsibility, even if the treatment was completely necessary? Will the insurance company cover the costs incurred by the patient? Should they take the loss or ask the patient to pay for a portion?

It's very easy to see which type of advocate you do not need, but it can be a challenge to decide the level of expertise you need once you decide you need a private professional patient healthcare advocate. More often than not, this is the kind of advocate who will serve your family best. Patients pay us directly, so our allegiance is to the patient and family alone.

What is a Private Professional Healthcare Advocate?

Private professional healthcare advocacy is a young but rapidly growing profession. In broad terms, a professional patient advocate is focused on three main priorities: quality care, preventing medical error, and protection of patient rights. Advocates can also save clients thousands of dollars when negotiating with insurance companies, not to mention saving lives and bringing peace of mind to families in crisis. Besides helping patients, professional advocates benefit hospitals by reducing readmissions, preventing medical error, and providing improved communication and education to families in medical need.

At the present time, advocates can come from many different walks of life and educational backgrounds. There are certificate programs in patient advocacy offered at a few large universities for people desiring to enter the field. Please do not misconstrue an advocate who has completed a *certificate program* at a university to mean that the advocate has taken a written *accreditation/ credentialing exam* that tests their knowledge and skills. There is presently no national accreditation examination for private patient advocates, though it is in the development stages now. We anticipate that the first testing will occur in 2018.

If you do an online search for patient advocacy, there are three main advocacy associations that will frequently appear. They are NAHAC, APHA, and PPAI.

Trisha Torrey founded APHA, or Alliance of Professional Health Advocates, in 2009. According to their website, the goal of APHA is "to help private, independent advocates start and grow successful practices, to help them maximize their reach, and therefore maximize patient success" (Alliance of Professional Health Advocates, 2016). They boast a membership of over 550 independent advocates. APHA has an online directory called AdvoConnection, where the public can search their database of members.

The National Association of Healthcare Advocacy Consultants (NAHAC) was also founded in 2009. NAHAC also has an online database of members, the *National Directory of Healthcare Consultants*, that the public can utilize when searching for an advocate. Here is what NAHAC has to say about their organization:

1. We promote rigorous standards for the practice of advocacy including ethical considerations and codes of conduct when providing medical decision-making support;

2. We educate consumers and healthcare professionals on research and current trends in patient-centered navigation, advocacy and decision-making support;

3. We partner with individual advocates and other grassroots organizations to collaborate on patient-centered reforms that maximize use of the healthcare system, protect consumer choice and improve access to high-quality, affordable care.

In 2009, NAHAC developed an Advocate Code of Ethics; I personally served as a member on the committee that wrote it. They also recently developed a set of recommendations called Best Practices and Standards that will be a first step in developing a national accreditation process. These guidelines were presented at the NAHAC conference held in Chicago in October 2014. The three main advocacy associations (NAHAC, PPAI, and APHA) collaborated to decide what qualifications should be required of professional patient advocates in the future as well as what the testing and national accreditation process will look like.

The Patient Advocacy Certification Board (PACB), the organization charged with developing a certification exam for patient advocates, summarizes the roles that patient advocates play in this way:

1. Provides services to patients as they navigate the healthcare system;

2. Works directly with patients to ensure that they have a voice in their care;

3. Works to make sure that patients have sufficient information to promote informed decision-making;

4. Plays an informational role;

5. Is committed to helping patients make informed choices and access resources;

6. Ensures that a patient's wishes are the guiding force behind decisions affecting medical care and the withholding of care; and

7. Collaborates effectively with other members of the healthcare team.

It is also important to understand what an advocate *cannot* do for you. The first ethical standard developed by NAHAC is very clear that advocates will not be the providers of direct medical care. It states that advocates "shall not recommend specific treatment choices, provide clinical opinions, or perform medical care of any type, even if they possess clinical credentials" (Patient Advocate Certification Board).

From my perspective as a nurse advocate, medically trained and experienced advocates are still the advocates of choice. A 2014 Gallup poll found that 80 percent of Americans believe that nurses have "very high" or "high" standards of honesty and ethics. Nurse advocates with strong clinical backgrounds are street-smart and savvy about where to go in hospitals to have our client's needs met. We review medical records and see red flags in charts that the average non-medical advocate would never catch. We know how to stand up for our clients and how to interact with medical professionals in a nonthreatening way to get what our client needs. We know the danger spots and we thoroughly understand patient rights. Typically, we are experienced as advocates from the onset because we have protected our own families and friends when they were going through healthcare crises as well.

While it's true that everyone needs an advocate, we have seen many different reasons that people do *not* hire an advocate when they are experiencing healthcare or elder care transitioning crises. The most common reason is that most people do not even know the industry exists — or what value we provide for patients and families.

The second-biggest reason is price. People are still in shock from all of the increased out-of-pocket expenses they are experiencing since the Affordable Care Act came into law. Everyone I know agrees that there is little that is affordable in this new healthcare landscape: higher costs for insurance, higher deductibles, fewer doctors and dentists who can take Medicaid patients, rising costs of healthcare, etc.

I get it. My own insurance premiums have skyrocketed in recent years, and the future looks dismal. I was asked recently on a business news TV program if I thought it was all a big scam by the insurance companies. I told them that I doubted it very much. When Blue Cross Blue Shield loses 1.5 billion dollars in one year, they have no choice: premiums **have** to rise! It now looks more favorable for BCBS in 2016; they are actually making a profit now that they and other insurers have adjusted to the ACA. Overall, though, this is a scary time for healthcare in America!

One of the most common family dynamics I see when parents start to fail is when one child (usually a daughter) has to step up and do all the caregiving: going to doctor's appointments, arranging those appointments, paying their bills, and managing all the problems that arise when parents age and insist upon living in their own home until they die, safety be darned. As the time commitments increase (while said daughter is trying to run her own family, job, etc.) she grows frustrated and stuffs her anger. She gets sarcastic about the other siblings who won't step up to help, and she does not realize that her burnout makes her appear strident and martyr-like. She alienates herself from the rest of the family, who cannot or will not step up to help. The daughter often complains that she suffers alone, that nobody is willing to help and that she has to do it all. To this woman, I say (with kindness!), "You don't have to do everything. You don't have to do it alone. It is *your* choice. Take care of yourself!" There is help available on many fronts, whether you have financial resources or not.

Aging parents often pay more attention to an outsider (especially a nurse) than the requests of their own children. They are afraid of appearing weak, of being treated like a child by their own children. The last time my dear father visited me in Chicago, he was 74 years old; a helpful flight attendant asked if he could help him get his bag out of the overhead compartment. My father retorted, "What do you think I am? Feeble or something?!" Our family laughed about that for years, though not to his face.

Our parents' pride hurts, even though they know deep down that they are failing and cannot stay in their own home alone forever. The thought of moving is frightening and overwhelming. They fear they will not have the money to afford a comfortable place. Often, they hope they will die suddenly and avoid the calamity altogether. But then there are consequences after the death: guilt, anger, and regrets that will haunt families for years.

There is help available. A wise advocate can help families walk through the complexities of choices, estate planning, financial strategies, and the various options for people with limited income. Yes, there is a cost to hire a private advocate—but what about the cost of missteps along the way, medical error, early infirmity, and the very real possibility of death brought about by accidents? What is the cost of losing our parents or loved ones before we have to?

Everyone has choices, different levels of financial abilities, and the possibility of family members willing to share the work. And then there is the willingness to ask for help. As I said earlier, there are no do-overs with our parents. Our family was lucky to have an ICU on that cruise ship in Belize, so we are now in our ninth extra year of having Papa with us. Was it worth it? Undoubtedly. Papa has been able to experience the joy of five extra grandchildren being born, and he is now the primary caregiver for his wife Ramona, whose health has since deteriorated. Family is important and it really does take a village to surround our aging parents with all they need. Professional advocates can seamlessly become a part of the village that is engaged to help keep our parents around and healthy for as long as possible.

Whether you learn to do the job yourself or hire a professional advocate, one thing is certain: everyone needs a health advocate these days! The U.S. healthcare system is quickly evolving. I know I can't fix a broken system alone—but I can use my years of clinical experience to help people navigate it as safely, efficiently and as economically as possible... one person at a time.

That's why I tell people I have the greatest job in the world. I can make things possible that people are unable to do on their own. I talk to the right people, ask the right questions, and stand up for what is right and fair. Someday I will grow old and feeble; I will need the kindness and skill of others to help me heal. I hope that someone will be there for me. This job, this amazing privilege of being a private professional healthcare advocate, is not really a job. It is a calling. I am hoping that when I get there, the healthcare system in this country will have undergone some healing of its own.

This is the story of an advocate who stepped in to help a family member determine if his aging mother's living situation was truly the best option for her. Her son didn't know what she needed. He wasn't sure how to help her. He contacted a nurse advocate for assistance, and ultimately decided that the clinical expertise on the end of the advocate was necessary for the complex care of his mother.

Mr. Smith contacted us to evaluate his 94-year-old mother. She lived in a senior housing development with a full-time caregiver, Mr. Smith, in the home. He said his mom had recently fallen, and he wanted to know if this was a safe situation. Should the family start looking for a skilled nursing facility?

Upon meeting her, I realized that, despite her physical limitations, this dear woman had a very clear wish to stay in her own home, with live-in caregivers to attend to her. All her friends lived in that building. Her bridge groups, and even her doctor, were in that same building. I could see that she got around quite well with her walker, and she was clearly competent to make her own decisions. I told her son that I felt this would be a much better living situation, and with some adjustments in her plan of care and a review of her medical plan with her physician, she would likely live a longer, happier, and even safer life in her own home for some time.

However, I noticed something alarming when I reviewed this woman's medication list: a surprising number of prescription medications whose side effects include dizziness, weakness, and loss of appetite. Overmedication of seniors is a serious health hazard and is particularly dangerous in cases where the person is seeing multiple doctors. In the rush of quick office visits, many doctors do not take the time to carefully review the entire medication list. And then there's the issue of professional courtesy: doctors are often hesitant to discontinue medications that another physician has prescribed. This particular woman was taking 14 medications, three of which were psychotropic drugs, though she denied any history of mental illness. I have seen far too many seniors fall and break a hip or sustain a fractured skull secondary to probable medication-related issues. Broken bones in the elderly often have tragic domino-effect deterioration in other systems. For those who are discharged from a hospital to a local rehabilitation facility, the risk of acquiring a hospital-related or nursing-home-related infection may cause a multitude of other health problems, and even result in death.

Most people who hire a PPHA are amazed at all the ways that we help not only the patient, but the family as well. Just as I have told my own family members: if a mom is able to stay at home with her children when they are young, it is a choice they will never live to regret. There are no do-overs with our children when they are young; we will never get those years back. The same is true with our parents. Though none of us has perfect parents, when they grow old and feeble, they need our help. If we can stop and put our own careers on hold to help them, and if we do that with great love, tenderness, and skill, we will never regret those years. Our own children will watch how we respect and value our parents, and that is how they will treat us when our time comes.

But for those adult children who are unable or unwilling to put their lives on hold to attend to their aging family member's needs, the next best thing (and often the better thing) is to hire a PPHA. An advocate will watch over their care, go to doctors' appointments, review their medical records, and if the client is admitted, a PPHA will go to the hospital, review the medical records, and ask all the tough questions. They will arrange for the right kind of home care services and even negotiate and resolve billing and insurance problems. Our clients tell us all the time that there has never been a time in U.S. history when our services are more needed, and I must agree after walking this path with family members many times before. Investments of time, money, and care as we help our parents age is some of the best-spent money a family will ever spend. There are no do-overs where family is concerned!

PPHAs are paid consultancy fees by the patient or their family, typically $125-$200 per hour, to work within the system to achieve better outcomes for their clients. Neither Medicare nor private insurance will cover the cost of advocates. Long-term care policies may reimburse for our services under the "RN care management" label. Each policy is different.

Tips to Equip: Find the perfect advocate for your needs

1. **Fees may be paid by the patient or their loved ones, but the "client" is the patient — regardless of who is paying the fees.** To tell the truth, we sometimes experience some degree of ethical tension when we are hired by adult children to watch over their aging parents. At our advocacy firm, our nurses are always careful to point out that our client may not be the one who pays the bill, but the focus of

everything we do is centered on the patient, the one who is experiencing healthcare challenges. In most cases, the entire family agrees on a plan of care and how we support the patient. There are also times that we must work hard towards a collaborative plan that will meet the multiple needs of the patient, as well as their family (who may be paying the bills). Be transparent with your prospective advocate. Ask how the needs of all involved will be met.

2. **Professional advocates vary in their educational background and training.** Always ask about their credentials and experience when you interview them. It's important to know what your needs are before you hire an advocate. Perhaps you need someone simply to negotiate with your insurance company to pay your medical bills. You may not need a nurse or physician to help you with that type of situation, but you will need someone who has experience with insurance appeals. Perhaps you need a physician or nurse with sharp clinical skills to oversee a medical crisis. Don't go looking for an advocate without a clear sense of what your family needs, and pay attention to your instincts when you meet the company representative. Ask about their experience with successfully advocating in situations similar to your own. Read the contract carefully before you sign. Be sure and ask for a quote for services that you feel may be bundled together. Ask any questions that you can think of beforehand. Some private advocates will work alongside you and teach you how to be a more effective advocate yourself, saving you time and money in the long run.

3. **There are also private advocates who are not in the medical field at all who call themselves private professional health advocates (PPHAs) — with questionable qualifications and very slick marketing campaigns.** Some advocates are strictly business/marketing people who will charge large monthly maintenance fees to cover "all of your healthcare needs," though they lack personal mentoring or physicians or nurses working alongside them who know what good healthcare looks like. Ask questions about experience and education! There is a difference between care managers and professional advocates: though professional nurse advocates can do complex care management tasks, care managers cannot always do effective advocacy. Nurse advocates have a wider scope of practice. Our businesses are not corporate; they are private, personal, and very relational. It's not just what we do that matters; it's how we make people feel when they have their own private nurse advocate watching over them. I have had clients tell me that hiring their own nurse advocate was the best gift their children ever gave them.

4. **You may find hospitals and insurance companies that offer the services of their own "advocates" free of charge.** Why hire your own advocate instead of relying upon the hospital's patient advocate? One word: *allegiance*. Hospital advocates work for the risk management department of hospitals. Their job is to smooth out complaints and keep the hospital from being sued. Risk managers show up when doctors leave sponges in patients during surgery or when patients' families complain about quality-of-care issues. They, too, get their paychecks from the hospital. Though they are great at handling small complaints and negotiating

bills when sincere errors have been made, risk managers and hospital-based advocates are there for one reason: to save the hospital millions of dollars per year in legal fees and to protect the hospital's public image. The same is true for insurance company employees who call themselves patient advocates. Their job is to promote positive relations with customers while saving their company millions by not paying for claims they don't have to. Follow the money; that's how you will find who is really advocating on your behalf.

If you choose to advocate for yourself or your loved one, it is important to be watchful, vigilant, and present when doctors visit. I tell all my clients how essential it is to have a small notebook handy so you can remember all of the questions you have for the nurse or doctor when you see them. Write everything down and keep notes on what different doctors tell you. Ask anything you wish, but be careful with how much time you spend — doctors often see around 20 patients per day, and they have electronic medical records, orders, and reading of tests to do as well. Show respect and appreciation for good care as often as you can.

The following chapter goes into detail about private professional healthcare advocates and the level of detailed care they provide. I have asked my dear friend Kate Curler to tell her story here, not only as a legal professional in the advocacy field, but also as a family member who found her voice in advocating for her parents. Kate is one of Chicago's finest legal patient advocates, and she does her best work in the halls of skilled nursing facilities in the Chicago area. Kate knows where the best and worst facilities are, and it is a high compliment if she moves one of her clients to the better ones. Kate is a friend, a valuable colleague, and a funny and engaging person who can make the most difficult situations manageable when she steps in to advocate.

Chapter 3

My Caregiving Journey *by Kate Curler*

My personal experience as a caregiver and advocate for my parents was a journey of over 10 years. This experience led me to realize the importance for caregivers to have a strong advocate, and led me to launch my business and continue to fight for my clients. I now have a law office which offers legal services to seniors, the disabled and their families, and provides advocacy services for my clients to get the best care in nursing homes as well as the best access to services and resources to go home. I also work closely with caregivers to put plans together for loved ones. I have a true passion for this work and love what I do.

My mother, Deborah Curler, was diagnosed with Type 1 (juvenile) diabetes at age four in 1952. At that time, her life expectancy was 50 years of age. She eventually lived to 64 years of age, but she struggled with health issues for her last decade. In 2003, I lived in northern California, but I decided to move closer to my parents in Bay City, Michigan. I got a job as a prosecutor in 2003 and moved to Chicago.

My parents came to visit me in Chicago; somehow my mother got *e. coli* (a normal bacterium in the gut, but toxic if it gets into the blood). She made it back to Bay City before she became ill, but she lay in a septic coma for weeks. I took a leave from my job and sat at her bedside with my father, Ronald Curler. After her doctors told us over and over that she would not survive, one morning she woke up.

Her condition was bad. She had nerve damage and could barely move her arms and legs. There was only one good rehabilitation center in Bay City and I desperately wanted her to go there. The discharge person at the hospital told me this was not possible, as my mother did not have insurance to cover her for this facility. I learned firsthand the importance of advocacy and not taking no for an answer when a loved one's life is at stake.

I clearly told the discharge person that her answer was not going to work for my mother, and that we needed to find a better solution. I wanted someone to call the insurance company, whether she made the call or I did, to get to a different answer. She suggested I go get a cup of coffee with my father and assured me that she would work on it. I wasn't sure if this was just a trick to get rid of us, but was pleasantly surprised that security did not escort us out. When I came back, a different solution had emerged. The insurance company was willing to pay for her stay as long as she improved. In the end, my mother and father worked very hard during the 17 weeks of inpatient and outpatient rehabilitation necessary for her recovery. Afterwards, my mother resumed all her activities of independent daily living.

In 2007, my mother had coronary surgery. Her heart was damaged from decades of diabetes. The hospital was unable to bring her out of anesthesia, and she lingered in a coma for days. At the end of that week, she was not able to walk or move her arms enough to feed herself independently. I took another leave from work, this time from the private law firm I started working for after her last coma. When she was discharged, my mother did not meet the medical criteria for the good rehabilitation center she had previously used. She ended up at a nursing home for rehabilitation — and a horrible one at that.

The first day, they mismanaged her food intake and insulin. She had a huge spike in blood sugar and she felt horrible. They took her for rehabilitation, but they only did some range of motion exercises with her and put her back in bed. My mother was only 59 years old, and I believed she would die there. She had worked too hard in her prior rehabilitation to have this happen now.

Again, I advocated for my mother and looked for a solution. I talked to the administration and told them this quality of care was not acceptable. I arranged for my father to monitor her blood sugar to help staff. I hired someone, a family friend and retired nurse, to assist in her care. Like my clients, I refused to let my mother be treated like any other person in that nursing home. I have learned that when a client of mine is treated like most residents in a nursing home, the care is usually horrible. I strive to have my clients treated like individuals; sometimes that means supplemental care in nursing homes. The person I hired to work with my mother got her up in the morning, made sure she was in the chair and had breakfast, and helped my father monitor her blood sugar. She also made sure my mother was back in her chair after rehab and took extra steps to help her walk and move around in the evenings. Within three and a half weeks, my mother returned home.

On the second day of the nursing home, I returned to my job (now at a private firm) and only visited my parents for vacations My father, however, was caring for my mother full-time and, like so many spousal caregivers, was stressed out and not caring for himself. In 2010, my father had an aneurysm in his aorta, which is often fatal. I rushed back to Bay City and settled in for another hospital stay. I had a great job, with a bonus and partner opportunities. The stress on my job was too great at this point, though, and I lost my job. Like too many American caregivers, I was forced to choose between caring for my family and focusing on my career. Against all odds, my father survived — but was legally blind due to strokes in his eyes. Again, I kicked into advocacy mode and took him (twice) to a top eye clinic in Ann Arbor, Michigan, using innovative solutions, like a homemade large print phonebook and a talking watch, to allow him to live independently.

I went back and forth between Chicago and Bay City, looking for work. I had been a divorce attorney, so I looked in that field but found nothing. I decided to work temporary jobs and move into the field of estate planning, probate, elder law, and guardianship. I did a lot of volunteer work and fought for my clients as I did for my parents. I utilized resources, advocated for my clients to be treated better, looked for creative solutions, and worked to treat my clients like autonomous individuals who deserve respect. I was told over and over that this wasn't really elder law; this was something more. My parents and I continued to struggle as my father had a heart valve replacement surgery in 2011; my mother, after being given the wrong dosages of a couple of medications and a horrible hospital stay where I was unable to get to Bay City fast enough to help, passed away in January 2012.

I realized that the business idea I had come up with — helping people whether traditional legal services are needed or not — would not work in a traditional law firm. I decided to stop looking for work with law firms. I stopped all temporary work, and I launched the Law Office of Kate Curler in January 2013. I had put in time with a great deal of volunteer groups for aging and disability in the Chicago area. That work also allowed me to form relationships with the best resources and facilities in the area.

I see myself as an advocate who just happens to be an attorney. I feel blessed to do the work I do every day. I don't see the work I do as a job; I see it as an opportunity. My work honors my mother's legacy. My work means that my mother's hard work and dedication to living the best and most independent life she could will result in that same life being lived by my clients, through her daughter's hard work and dedication.

Chapter 4

The Sandwich Generation

We hear more and more about the Sandwich Generation: those who are caring for their children while also tending to aging parents.

The Sandwich Generation supersedes the Baby Boomers and Generation X because it includes all people with a parent over 65 who are also raising a child under 18 or financially supporting a child over 18. According to the 2013 Pew Research Study, 47 percent of people, aged 40-59 are members of the Sandwich Generation. (Pew Research Center, 2013)

When we think of people aged 40-59, we typically think of someone at the height of their career, working full-time, trying to pay their bills, and providing for their children (or paying for college if their kids are over 18) while hopefully planning for their retirement. Along with the adults' work, their kids may be heavily involved in sports or other activities that take up much of their free time. There is also an increase in chronic medical and developmental issues with children born in the last 10 years. Scientists report that one in 68 children born in the U.S. today will be diagnosed with autism (Centers for Disease Control, 2016). Add in the increasing numbers of children with life-threatening allergies and asthma, and many Sandwich Generation parents have children with complex medical issues that require additional care, time, and financial resources.

Now let's look at the aging parent side of the sandwich. They too may require financial assistance, emotional support, and extra care. According to the Pew study (Pew Research Center, 2013), around 15 percent of middle-aged adults are providing financial support to their children and parents simultaneously, while 73 percent of middle-aged adults surveyed by Pew have provided financial assistance to their children over 18. We hear about these issues all the time with our clients: for her safety, Mom really needs to move to a memory care facility, but it costs $9,000 a month and Medicare won't cover it. Dad desperately needs a new set of hearing aids, but they cost $5,000. The family house is 50 years old and needs a new roof, water heater, and furnace, but there is not enough money while paying for the nursing home. With people living longer, the costs associated with aging can be out of reach for many. Adult children can be caught in the middle, trying to pay their own bills and help their parents out financially at the same time. Pew found that 75 percent of respondents felt it an obligation to help their parents financially if they needed it.

We cannot discount the time we need to spend with our children as well as our aging parents. Pew notes that 68 percent of people aged 40-59 reported that their parents "frequently" or "sometimes" needed emotional support. Adding to the stress, 76 percent reported that their own adult children also needed support frequently or sometimes (Pew Research Center, 2013).

Assistance with day-to-day living is a huge issue. 28 percent of middle-aged adults below the age of 60 reported one or both parents needing help with daily living; 31 percent reported performed most of the assistance themselves, while 48 percent said they performed some of the assistance. When respondents to Pew's study were 60-years-old or greater, 50 percent of them reported a parent requiring day-to-day assistance (Pew Research Center, 2013). Caregivers are expensive and hard to find; who will foot the bill? And in the case of hospitalization, the pressures are even greater as the adult child tries to balance caring for their parent at the hospital, talking to their doctors, and trying to glean information from the medical jargon. All the while they shuttle the kids to and from school and they hope the boss will forgive the unplanned absence from work or decreased work performance. Many adult children end up losing their jobs due to increasing demands of caregiving spent on aging parents. I believe this generation is one of THE most stressed out groups of people in America today. Living with constant fear and anxiety affects adult children's health, their jobs, their families, and their quality of life.

When a parent's health fails, it is not uncommon for people to feel great stress and a loss of control, and we often see coping mechanisms that do not make sense at first glance. But the impending loss of a parent is a major life crisis, and people are often surprised when otherwise normal family members begin to act out, either by becoming hyper-controlling, emotionally distant, passive-aggressive, or overly angry towards other family members. It is important to step back and remain calm, especially when important decisions need to be made as a family unit. Each family member should remain respectful of others and keep their dignity at all times; momentary lapses in self-control with one's words may have far-reaching consequences, not only for the present generation but for future ones as well. Children tend to repeat family patterns, so please remember that your family will carefully watch your example. Ultimately, we are judged not for our intentions, but by our actions and words.

Years of ICU experience around the country have taught me, among other things, that when family members behave badly in public, it is usually because they are more afraid than angry. Anger is a secondary emotion. The primary one is fear.

Fear of losing a loved one can look different to each person, even in the same family unit. Birth order may be an important factor in how each one deals with death and dying, as well. Previous losses and experiences with death also play a factor in how one grieves—or does not grieve—in the present moment. Certainly there's no one right way to grieve, but since everyone does handle loss differently, it's important to be patient with others, just as you should be gentle with yourself.

I have found that listening is the most important thing that healthcare professionals and family members can do when confronted with an angry, emotionally distraught, or grieving person. If the anger has a just cause, the problem can often be addressed and resolved. If, however, the anger and lashing out at others is generalized, it may be a sign of great pain and can only be resolved through kindness, compassion, and a sincerely caring ear. It's hard to find in today's fast-paced world, but it is critically necessary. I remind myself often that the anger is not about me — it is because anger is much easier for people to deal with than grief. Anger feels powerful. Admitting to deep grief and sadness makes people feel vulnerable, incapable and lost. Simply being there for someone in deep pain is more important than most people realize. We are a blanket of protection and safety, helping not only the patient/client, but the entire family as well. Every week I hear from family members who are stressed, burned out, and frustrated with managing everything on their own. I wish we could help more people who are struggling, but everyone must decide what value is when dealing with these complex issues. Unfortunately, we often see people who have (unintentionally, of course) made an absolute mess of things before they call us in.

Tips to Equip: Assistance for the Sandwich Generation

1. **Ask the village for help!** It takes a village to raise a child. Befriend other parents who can help out with driving to baseball practice or transport to birthday parties. With 47 percent of adults in the Sandwich Generation, chances are good that there are fellow parents out there who will understand your need for help (and will probably ask for your help, too!). Pay the neighbor's kid to mow the lawn while you spend some time catching up with your spouse. Take care of your bill-paying electronically, and schedule automatic payments so you don't find yourself with late charges.

2. **Take care of yourself, even in small ways, as often as you can.** Sandwich Generation adults can find themselves not eating properly, not exercising, and not taking time for themselves. While you may not have time for the gym membership, you can park the car further at work and get some extra steps in—or you can meet up with a friend and walk and talk on your lunch break. Mindfully choose healthier, yet still simple meals. There are many great options today, even at quick restaurants, if you don't have time to prepare a meal. Find hair salons that will cut your kids' hair at the same time you get yours cut.

3. **Talk to someone.** If you find yourself stressed out, feeling sad, or not sleeping well, help can be a phone call away. If dear friends are also busy like you, there are website

therapists who will Skype with you over the phone, rather than insisting you drive to their office. If you're affiliated with a church, talking with a respected clergy member can help as well. Everyone needs help sometimes, and there should be no shame in asking for it.

4. **Consult with a private professional healthcare advocate (PPHA).** A PPHA can do a wide variety of things to help you keep your parents healthy and safe. They can help manage your parents' medical care, facilitate communication between physicians, organize medication management, and suggest devices that will make living on their own easier and safer. They can help you get all your medical affairs in order so that when you need help quickly, costly medical error is avoided. If you're not sure, a PPHA can help assess whether seniors are safe to live on their own; or they can suggest high-quality senior living communities that are within their budget. They can also help you navigate the complex world of Medicare and insurance concerns, and they can refer you to other high-quality specialists who can help you manage your loved ones' care.

Chapter 5

The Patient Bill of Rights: Don't Leave Home Without It!

Do you know your rights as a patient — from a legal standpoint?

Your rights go well beyond the HIPAA (Health Insurance Portability and Accountability Act) laws governing the privacy of your personal information.

This chapter highlights the value a PPHA can add to your healthcare experience, especially in helping you *exercise* your rights.

It may seem like a lot of mumbo-jumbo, but knowing the law regarding your rights is crucial to your survival. You must ensure that you are well informed, and that you receive the proper treatment to improve your quality of life from a healthcare perspective.

After you finish reading this chapter, you will be prepared to advocate on your own behalf — and you will be prepared to recognize if the private professional healthcare advocate you have chosen to carry out your wishes is up to the task.

Even if you don't remember the law, word-for-word, as it relates to your rights, the information in this section will help you become familiar enough to know when something is not right — or if you feel something is being overlooked.

You've probably overlooked the large banner posted in almost every hospital you've ever visited. It is titled: PATIENT BILL OF RIGHTS. It's usually prominently posted in a main hallway of the hospital. Because it is so unobtrusive, you may look at it, but not really *see* it.

That poster is chock-full of valuable information that can help you navigate your way through a hospital stay, be it an unexpected procedure the doctor wants you to have right away or your right to know more about a test you're unsure of, your right to request a second opinion, and a host of other privileges you're entitled to simply because you are the patient. In fact, even the medical record itself is the legal property of the patient. No hospital can deny you access to that record. After this section, you'll never pass that poster again without looking twice.

William's story will be shared later on in this chapter; his rights as a patient were violated by well-meaning hospital staff without perspective. Advocates are important in telling the entire story to healthcare providers! When an advocate understands hospital hierarchy, issues with liability, and can speak in medical language — all while avoiding going to court — it is a win for everyone.

Exercising your rights are only possible when you know your rights! Many versions of a Patient Bill of Rights have been circulated over the years, but the U.S. House and Senate have never passed official legislation to adopt one.

In 2003, the American Hospital Association revised their original Patient Bill of Rights, and the AHA document formerly known as the Patient Bill of Rights was revised and shortened and is now known as the Patient Care Partnership. The AHA publishes a pamphlet bearing the same name;

ideally it would be given to patients at the beginning of their stay, although when casually surveyed, we couldn't find a patient who has ever seen this pamphlet.

Here are the tenets of The Patient Care Partnership taken straight from the brochure (*American Hospital Association*):

1. **High quality hospital care.** You have the right to medical care provided with "skill, compassion, and respect." In turn, you have the obligation to inform your caregivers if you are in pain or you have concerns about your care.

2. **A clean and safe environment.** Clean and safe are broad terms. The AHA dictates that hospitals will use policies and procedures to keep you safe, and that if an "unexpected and significant" event occurs, you will be informed of it as well as any changes in your care as a result. More on this in a following chapter: *Dangers Lurking in Every Hospital.* "Clean" in my world means no contact with hospital infections, but that can only be avoided by staying out of hospitals altogether.

3. **Involvement in your care.** This is a broad subject broken down by the AHA into the following subsets:

   - **Getting information from you.** In order for the hospital to provide proper treatment, you need to be open and honest about your past illnesses, surgeries, hospitalizations, past allergic reactions, and any medications and dietary supplements (vitamins and herbs) you may be taking. You also need to inform them of your insurance status as well as any network or admission requirements that your insurance may have.

- **Understanding your healthcare goals and values.** You have the obligation to inform your doctor, your care team, and your family of your healthcare goals and values. The hospital will consider those values throughout your hospital stay. Ideally, they should ask you what your goals are every day.

- **Discussing your medical condition and information about appropriate treatment choices.** When you and your doctor discuss treatment choices, you should be involved. You have the right to understand the various treatment options along with their risks and benefits, whether the treatment is proven or experimental (in clinical trials), and what long-term side effects and/ or benefits you should expect from the treatment. You and your family have the right to know what needs to be done to take care of you after you leave the hospital. This extends into financial issues too; you have the right to understand the financial ramifications of receiving services not covered by your insurance, or using out-of-network medical providers. If you are a senior who is admitted under observation status, a care manager should sit down with you, explain the financial ramifications of that, and have you sign a MOON (Medicare Outpatient Observation Notice) document. You have the obligation to tell your medical providers if you need more information about your treatment choices.

- **Discussing your treatment plan.** You have the right to consent to or refuse a treatment plan. If you refuse a treatment, your doctor should explain the consequences of refusing. You also have the right to participate, or refuse to participate, in a clinical research study.

- **Understanding who should make decisions when you cannot.** If you already have legal documents, such as a healthcare power of attorney, please inform your doctor, your care team, and your family. If you need help in making difficult decisions, the hospital will have on hand a social worker and/or chaplain to assist you. Living wills and other lay documents do not carry the full weight that power of attorney for healthcare documents do. If people come in without a POA, the hospital has to guess who the surrogate decision-maker should be if the person becomes incapacitated in any way. Every person over the age of 18 should have a healthcare POA document; hospital staff need to know who has legal rights to information as well as decision-making power. If you do *not* want to be resuscitated for any reason, you will need to have a POLST (Physician's Order for Life-Sustaining Treatment) form signed and witnessed.

- **Protection of your privacy.** Hospitals are mandated under HIPAA (Health Insurance Portability and Accountability Act) law to respect and protect the confidentiality of your relationship with your doctors and other caregivers, as well as all sensitive information about your health. State and federal laws, as well as hospital policies, protect the privacy of your medical information. You will receive a native of Privacy Practices that describes the way your care providers use, disclose, and safeguard patient information upon hospital admission, and it explains how you can obtain a copy of your medical records. In practice, with wireless cloud-sharing between hospitals, it is easy for people not involved with your care to obtain private information. It is difficult to monitor that activity; however, care providers understand the law and do their best to protect it. Sometimes it is hard to get access to needed information that you as the patient have a right to view (or would want shared with your family or an advocate when requested), because healthcare providers misunderstand its practical application. For more information about what HIPAA really means, please check out the AHA's letter to Health and Human Services Secretary Kathleen Sebelius; it is titled "The HIPAA Privacy Rule Accounting of Disclosures." The HITECH (Health Information Technology for Economic and Clinical Health) Act is worth reading up on as well. The Department of Health and Human Services has helpful information on their website at **HHS.gov** or **CMS.gov**.

- **Help with your bill and filing insurance claims.** The American Hospital Association is staffed with helpful and friendly insurance experts who will guide you through the process of filing claims and will be available for any questions you may have. They offer help in finding financial aid and payment plans, as well as other ways of managing your hospital debt.

- **Preparing you and your family for when you leave the hospital.** The AHA's brochure states, "You can expect us to help you identify sources of follow-up care and to let you know if our hospital has a financial interest in any referrals. As long as you agree that we can share information about your care with them, we will coordinate our activities with your caregivers outside the hospital."

High-quality hospital care. The AHA emphasizes being treated with skill, compassion, and respect. A chilling piece of insider info: if you are admitted through the emergency room without your own admitting physician, you will be assigned to the physician on call for the day. You read that right: it is purely luck (good or bad) if you leave your choice of physicians up to the hospital. Most physicians no longer see their own patients while they're in the hospital; in the case of hospitalization you will be assigned a hospitalist to oversee your care. A hospitalist is a physician who is employed by the hospital to take care of hospitalized patients. While they may be very knowledgeable, they do not know you or your medical history, other than what you can provide. Fragmented care at its worst and most dangerous is having a complete stranger take care of you at your very sickest. Ask most primary care physicians how they feel about not being allowed to manage their own patients in the hospital; they do not want their patients managed by strangers either. Sometimes the doctors are not even notified when their patient is admitted!

Take hope: your involvement in your own care will ultimately improve the quality of the healthcare you receive, no matter whom you receive it from. Many hospitalists are fine clinicians with excellent skills; they just do not have the long-term relationship and the allegiance that the patient's own doctor has for each patient, nor do they know what each patient's "normal" looks like. You are obliged to provide accurate information regarding your diet; your alcohol and tobacco habits; your symptoms and any medications, vitamins, and supplements that you take; past medical and surgical history; and the different doctors that you see. A private healthcare advocate can gather this information for you and create a personalized medical profile for you to bring to all of your doctor's appointments. Having the correct information will help you get the most out of your appointments and will improve the quality of your care. I have accompanied many of our clients to the ED over the past six years, and I almost always hear statements like, "This is great! May I copy this?" or "What a time saver this is!" from care providers. Talking with another healthcare professional about the patient's medical history saves time, prevents medical errors, and gets the patient diagnosed and treated much faster.

Many patients are reluctant to tell their physician absolutely everything out of fear of being judged; a frequent example is admitting alcohol use. Patient J routinely drinks six cans of beer after work every day, but he tells his doctor that he has two beers every Saturday night. When Patient J lands in the hospital after a car accident, the hospital physician is unaware that Patient J is a routine drinker, and after two days in the hospital Patient J goes into alcohol withdrawal (delirium tremens, or DT's), has multiple seizures, and ends up in the intensive care unit on life support. Alcohol withdrawal is no laughing matter! Doctors need to know the truth, so they can diagnose and treat early if patients start to go into withdrawal. Patients in DT's can become violent, hallucinate, and even seize, so hospital personnel need to be prepared.

You have an obligation to share your health goals and values with your healthcare team as well as your family. This can be difficult, because you may have vastly different goals than your healthcare team or than what your family wishes for you.

An example: Patient Y has just been diagnosed with liver cancer. Her family doctor, after looking at her CT scan reports, gives a grim prognosis, but sends her off to see the oncologist all the same. The oncologist develops a chemotherapy plan and seems optimistic. The family is thrilled that the oncologist is so enthusiastic, and they are angry at the family physician for being so negative. The truth is, Patient Y trusts and believes her family physician, and doesn't want to proceed with the chemo but does so because of her oncologist's encouragement and her family's expectations. Patient Y decides that she will only agree to chemotherapy in pill form. She takes the pills for a few days and develops side effects that land her in the hospital with severe bleeding, requiring multiple blood transfusions. After five days in the hospital, she declares to her doctor and her family that she will never return to the hospital for any reason. She engages in-home hospice services and dies peacefully two weeks later, comfortable and surrounded by her loved ones. I cannot stress the importance of thoughtful, careful consideration of any treatment plan your doctor offers, strongly enough. Just because a doctor strides confidently into a patient's room and declares what "we" are going to do, it does not mean it is the right thing to do. It's the patient's body and their life. The patient should ALWAYS be well-informed about their diagnosis, treatment options, and potential for any adverse side effects or risks involved.

William's Story

Two years ago, William was a 48-year-old engineer living by himself when he fell off a ladder while changing a light bulb in his kitchen. As he fell, the back of his neck landed sharply on the edge of his kitchen counter — just like that, William became a quadriplegic. One of his sisters found him and he was transferred to Chicago, to a major healthcare institution specializing in acute neurological injuries. He received good care initially, but over the course of the following year, he was in and out of 14 hospitals, long-term care facilities, and rehabilitation centers. During that period, William suffered from multiple infections, bed sores, incidents of respiratory failure, and pneumonia. He lost over 35 pounds, developed more infections and was on multiple antibiotics, which eventually resulted in bouts of sepsis from drug-resistant super-infections.

His sisters contacted us last year in desperation. They were afraid he was going to die. They had watched his gradual decline and they knew they had to do something, so they hired a PPHA. They were frustrated and angry at the insurance company, who kept mandating that he be transferred to low-quality skilled nursing facilities. When we met William, he had a tracheostomy, a feeding gastronomy tube, a catheter, a colostomy, and four large bed sores requiring wound vacuum therapy. He was on a respirator and was covered head-to-toe with severe rashes and flaking skin. His arms and legs were severely contracted and he was in an isolation room for a drug-resistant infection. Though he could not talk, his eyes lit up when he met us and we communicated nonverbally for half an hour. Our presence brought hope to William and his sisters, and they agreed to take a leap of faith in hiring us to advocate in a way that they had been unable to do.

Over the next six weeks, we met regularly with the care manager at his rehab facility to make arrangements for him to come home. The sisters, as well as William himself, knew he would be able to receive the best care at home from people who knew and loved him. As a former ICU nurse, I knew what could be accomplished at home with the right support, and we persevered through many obstacles to get him home. I think the facility staff thought we had all lost our marbles to imagine that we could take such a complex patient home, but his family was determined and we knew we could make it work.

The day came for William to come home and I arrived at his home first to make certain that his equipment had arrived and was functioning properly: much to my dismay, the nursing home care manager had hired a substandard medical supply company and his hospital bed and air mattress were inadequate to ensure that his skin did not break down further. By this point I had developed a working relationship with the insurance company's RN case manager, so I was able to explain all the danger to her and appeal for a much higher-quality bed. This request was granted, and William thrived at home for the next 18 months, receiving excellent care from his family and a wonderful live-in caregiver who treated him like a beloved family member. Unfortunately, before the new high-tech bed arrived, after the initial hospitalization, our client ended up back in a local hospital due to wound narcosis, caused by an inadequate air mattress on his bed. At that time, he required surgery to have the would surgically altered, so the health tissue could again begin to heal.

One thing lead to another, and poor infection control practices and sloppy care resulted in multiple complications; pneumonia, due to lack of sterile techniques during suctioning and anemia due to antibiotics that required 10 units of blood to be transfused over one month, and severe anxiety and pain resulting from the adverse medical outcomes that we observed.

Everything was documented and brought to the attention of the hospital staff in a calm, professional manner. Our client's sister was aghast at the lack of infection control measures she observed and was desperate to get her brother out of the hospital. After three weeks, he came home to a brand-new ICU "Cadillac" bed that continually, slowly, rotated him from side to side. The bed had to be specially requested through corporate administration due to the cost: $48,000 retail. It has helped William heal at home, prevent pneumonia occurrences, and also save wear and tear on his family members' backs. They no longer have to wake up in the night to turn him every two hours. The bed has been instrumental in keeping him home, healthy, and happy. Twice weekly, skilled nursing visits are paid for by his insurance company and we stay in close contact with his family, helping to avoid needless hospitalizations by intervening early when small problems occur.

When William came back home after his last hospital nightmare, I decided to pay a friendly call to the hospital's risk management department. I politely relayed the things we had observed that were clearly against any hospital's infection control policies. I told them that I had no intention of advising the family to seek legal counsel. But, I said, we also sincerely hoped that this gentleman would receive no bill from the hospital, since three unfortunate instances of medical error had been observed and documented. Our client has never received a bill in the past year since this hospitalization occurred. We were able to save between $5,000-$10,000 in non-covered medical bills.

After 18 months of living at home with no infections and a much-improved quality of life, William developed an unexpected leak of cerebrospinal fluid, which led to a bad case of pneumonia, and another hospitalization. Once again, the problems began and over the course of the next year, he developed even worse strains of multi-drug resistant, nosocomial infections. Nosocomial essentially means "acquired in the hospital," is one of the main reasons why we wanted to keep him out of there: too many germs and a weakened immune system on his part, made worse by a nonstop onslaught of stress, pain, poor nutrition, and an avalanche of powerful antibiotics over months and years.

A few months ago, I got another phone call from one of his sisters: "Teri, we need you back again. They don't want William to come home and we're afraid he's going to die if we let them send him to another nursing home."

Two days later, I took the ten hour trip to the long-term acute care hospital where he was being treated. His family told me he was on the ventilator and that staff had tried to wean him off several times unsuccessfully. When I saw him, he was on simple humidified oxygen to his tracheostomy and he was in no distress at all. I learned that the medical team was putting him back on the respirator every night, which I suspected was for the staff's convenience more than for the patient's benefit. He had recently been transferred to the main hospital after developing an airway obstruction from not being suctioned as often as he needed it. I was shocked to hear that he sometimes had to wait 20-40 minutes for someone to answer his call light. He was in intensive care. When I worked in ICU, the standard was always less than three minutes *at the very most* to attend a patient on a ventilator who needed help. His sister told me of other incidences where the facts of his case had been misrepresented.

When I spoke to his insurance nurse case manager, I learned that she was in the Acceleration department of the company. This man no longer met the criteria for a LTACH (long-term acute care hospital) and he was being advised to go to a nursing home that could care for his needs properly (the ventilator and the many tubes and wounds). Unfortunately, the quality facilities with that level of experience would not accept him due to the complexity of his infection.

When I discussed his case at length with the insurance company case manager, I listed the many reasons why he would be better off at home: two full-time caregivers so he would never have to wait to be suctioned again; no hospital environment ripe for more infections; a trained, devoted sister who knew how to skillfully and cleanly care for his tracheostomy, feeding tube, colostomy and wounds; and a special care bed much better than the standard-issue hospital bed. He would be happier, healthier and more comfortable in his own home!

After listing every medical reason why I knew he would be better off at home, I also informed her that he would have two advanced-practice RNs on 24-hour care for him; a home health RN skilled at complex wound care; and a home visiting physician who knew the family well. Lastly, I pointed out that the insurance company would save money by getting him out of a facility that was costing the insurance company at least $7,000 per day. Her excitement was palpable; she urged me to move full steam ahead and she would approve anything we needed to get him home. The medical establishment was not so easy to convince. They called for an ethics committee meeting. I enthusiastically agreed, knowing that I would have a full and impartial audience to make my case.

The following Wednesday, I arrived with my complete medical profile, care plan and supporting documents. I was asked to wait in the hallway until they were ready... twenty minutes later. I thought that was odd; there is not supposed to be a "meeting before the meeting" on ethics committee hearings. When they finally admitted me, I saw that they had, in fact, not invited any impartial committee members. Just twelve of them from the hospital — and me.

William's sisters had declined the chance to attend, since they felt that their emotions may get out of hand. They trusted me to represent their case well. I had talked to them about what they would and would not go along with, if a compromise became necessary. I knew the staff was going to tell me that he could only go home if he was discharged to hospice, under palliative care. My ace in the hole was a company in Illinois I found that would admit him under palliative care only, with no Do Not Resuscitate order required. It was *not* hospice, though the parent company did have both hospice and palliative care divisions. They did not require a DNR order, as most hospice companies do.

During the ethics committee meeting, I first assured them that I was a career ICU nurse and I understood their hesitation in sending a patient with so many complex health issues home. I told them that the family had hired me instead of an attorney because medical advocates know more about healthcare and patients' rights than most attorneys. I was there to prevent this case from requiring legal action.

I know that part of the mounting costs of U.S. healthcare is due to far too many malpractice suits. It drives up the cost of healthcare for all of us. I listened to them, I answered their concerns, and I laid out my plan just as I had with the insurance company. I gave them a complete list of all 22 different facilities he had been in over the past three years. I listed the many complications, incidences of medical error, and infections to which he had been victim. One facility had even broken his hip during a physical therapy session! I listed every reason why his family and I believed, with all our hearts, that he would be safer and better cared-for at home. I told them about the stress his sisters had been under with the nonstop trauma over the past three years. I explained why they had good, fact-based reasons not to trust the medical establishment.

As the meeting went on, I saw some of them begin to soften. The head of the ethics committee actually had some hospice experience and was familiar with the palliative care company I mentioned. When the doctor told me they would only agree to discharge if he went to a palliative/hospice company, I explained that the patient and family did not want to receive hospice services, but would agree to palliative with a full CODE order for pain management only. I could see that we had found a loophole.

Another doctor seemed angry that I was there to oppose his plan, which was to transfer him to a skilled nursing facility. The doctors saw William's case as a massive liability; doctors fear lawsuits more than anything, so they were cautious. I told him that I could not, in good conscience, suggest any of the awful facilities on the short list that would even accept him. He was disqualified from the better facilities because of the infection that this hospital had given my client. We simply had no better choice than sending him home.

Since I knew the home environment and support he would have, I hoped that I had ultimately allayed the doctor's concerns. But this particular doctor was still unhappy. He told me, "You are his advocate! It is your job to be honest with him and tell him he will die if he goes home!"

I reminded him that I was the patient's advocate, not the hospital's, nor the insurance company's advocate, and that I served the patient only. I would not have driven two and a half hours that day to address the ethics committee if I did not completely agree with my client and his family. "Besides," I told him, "even if he is ultimately going to die early from his condition, shouldn't he have the *right* to say where he will live out the rest of his days? Isn't it his *right to choose* where he lives and dies?"

Silence blanketed the room for a moment. Then the head of the ethics committee, a physician, stood up, shook my hand and said, "Okay! Let's get him home!" There were smiles and handshakes all around after that, and I left very pleased. We had won. It was a good day.

I later discovered the reason why no outside members of the ethics committee were in attendance that day. The hospital did not want impartial witnesses to be present at the meeting. The chief nursing officer took the meeting notes. Afterwards, there was a "meeting after the meeting" to decide what to document. They documented things that were patently untrue and claimed that I agreed to have the family sign William out against medical advice. An AMA document opens up the family to be liable for costs not covered by insurance, and the insurance company had told the hospital weeks before that he would not be covered.

I had never experienced a hospital ethics committee actually *lying* before, but I figured they must have been desperate to protect their reputation and their perceived liability. I let this go, and chalked it up to one more lesson learned about the way modern healthcare works today. My job is to protect and advocate for my client's welfare. We had won our case, and that's all that really mattered. We still had several battles to fight before he came home. Fortunately, he did come home within a week and we all sighed with relief. I'm sure the doctors and nurses at the facility had never seen such a complex patient being sent home before, but the advances in home healthcare management have made it possible to do things today that couldn't have been done even ten years ago. With the right support, including two standby advanced practice nurse advocates on 24-hour call for William, as well as the rest of our team, we knew he would be better off; he would live longer and he would avoid more of the infections and medical error that had already happened to him.

In this case, perseverance for patient rights paid off!

Tips to Equip: Take action if you aren't being treated with skill, compassion, and respect

1. **Trust your instincts.** We humans usually have a good sense of when things aren't going as they should. It's difficult to speak up when you're in a hospital bed. If possible, ask a friend or a loved one to be at your bedside, especially in the early mornings when most doctors make their rounds.

2. **Speak to your nurse about your concerns.** Nurses usually know the individual physicians quite well, and they may be able to give you insight or intercede on your behalf.

3. **Try to discuss and explain your issues as calmly and**

kindly as you can. That old adage is true; you always catch more flies with honey than vinegar.

4. **You or a loved one should document your experiences on paper.** Include dates, times, and names.

5. Many hospitals have their own "advocates" who are employees whose sole purpose is to keep patients happy, so they don't end up suing them later on. **Ask for the advocate to come to your room and see if they can help you.** Ask about their credentials: often hospital advocates are not even nurses; they act as customer service representatives without any real knowledge of what a problem entails from a medical perspective. A nurse advocate at the hospital is better than no advocate at all.

6. If you have the courage and are feeling up to it, you could **address the physician directly,** or have a loved one address them for you.

7. If those measures don't work? **Ask for the "charge nurse" in your unit.** That is the nurse who is overseeing all the nurses for that day.

8. **You can always request a different physician.** There is usually more than one hospitalist on duty. This may be challenging, due to doctors protecting their colleagues, but you can ask.

9. If you don't get anywhere with the charge nurse? Go up the chain and **ask for the nursing supervisor;** this is the nurse in charge of the nurses all over a particular hospital unit.

10. The final approach is to **ask your nurse for the phone number to risk management**. This is the department in the hospital that handles lawsuits and potential lawsuits. Oftentimes just asking for their number will get you somewhere in the right direction.

Tips to Equip: Get involved in your care!

1. **Not many patients question their doctor's treatment plan, but everyone should.** Treatment plans can be complicated and difficult to understand. There may be more than one treatment option available, and you should understand all of them. A private advocate with medical training can do a lot to advance your understanding of your treatment options. If an advocate isn't available to you, bring a loved one or a friend to listen and take notes; it is difficult to take all the information in when you're thinking about your medical concerns!

2. **Clinical trials may be an option.** A clinical trial occurs after a drug or device has been tested in a lab setting. There are different phases of clinical trials, which indicate how far along the medication or device has been studied and tested. Doctors have to work with the Food and Drug Administration (FDA) on clinical trials; they cannot just decide to invent a new drug, procedure, or device and try it out themselves. There is a definite process involved. Some clinical trials go very well, and new technology or medications become available to the public as a result. Other clinical trials are a disaster—patients die or have severe complications—and the FDA calls a halt to the whole trial.

- Please don't discount the options of clinical trials; sometimes they may be your best, or only, chance at improvement. Patients can often be fragile, and their bodies simply cannot undergo a surgery that is routinely recommended for their condition. An example: a woman had a severely leaky valve in her heart. She desperately needed a replacement valve, but that would mean open-heart surgery and her heart was just too weak to undergo it. The doctor mentioned a clinical trial of a valve replacement that didn't involve sawing her chest open. It was still risky, due to its experimental nature and the routine risks of anesthetic use, but it was a much shorter anesthetic time and a much easier recovery without opening the chest cavity. It was a tremendous success, and the woman made an excellent recovery and returned to a great quality of life.

- We hear a lot about clinical trials for cancer drugs. When a patient has run out of options for treatment, they may decide to enroll in a clinical trial. The drug may help them, and they will help others as well by allowing themselves to be part of the study.

3. **Don't forget that you do have the right to refuse recommended treatment.** A woman went to her gynecologist for some abnormal bleeding. The doctor mentioned a hysterectomy to remove her uterus; that was all the patient heard. She signed the consent forms for the surgery, put a date on the calendar, and came back to her doctor for her pre-operative physical. She cried to the medical assistant, "I don't want to have a hysterectomy, but he [the doctor] says I have to." The medical assistant shared the patient's concerns with the physician, and the

surgery was immediately cancelled. The doctor prescribed some medications to help the bleeding. Fortunately, the patient had the courage to tell the medical assistant her concerns about the surgery, and fortunately the medical assistant shared her concerns with the physician. In that moment, the medical assistant was a healthcare advocate.

Refusing treatment doesn't mean your physician is going to agree with you, and they will probably do their best to talk you out of it if they feel it is not a good idea, but it is ultimately your decision. It's your body, after all! Emergency department physicians can relate many stories of patients who are brought in by ambulance (usually after another person has called the ambulance), found to be having a heart attack and yet—for reasons of their own—they refuse treatment. As long as this patient has stable vital signs and a normal oxygen level, they appear to be thinking clearly, and are not intoxicated, they are usually allowed to refuse treatment after they sign an AMA form, shorthand for leaving the hospital "against medical advice." We, as nurses and doctors, may not agree with their opinion, and we do our best to inform and educate, but ultimately it is the patient's choice. On more than one occasion, those patients have been brought back to the hospital after suffering a full cardiac arrest at home. Also important to know: if a patient signs out AMA, the insurance company has the right to refuse to pay the bill in most cases, so the patient may be liable for thousands of dollars' worth of healthcare expenses. It is almost *never* a good idea to sign out AMA just because you disagree with the doctors. Go up the chain of command and try your best to resolve the dispute, or hire an advocate to fight on your behalf.

Here are some instances in which you will *NOT* have the right to refuse treatment:

1. **You are a non-pregnant minor.** Pregnant minors are in a tricky and confusing situation. They can make decisions for their unborn child and they can make pregnancy-related decisions, such as consenting to an abortion. The pregnant minor, however, cannot make other medical decisions for themselves. For example, a pregnant minor cannot sign a consent form for an appendectomy. Their parent still has to sign for any non-pregnancy-related conditions. To muddy the waters further, a teenage parent can sign for their own child's appendectomy (or other surgery), but they cannot sign for their own appendectomy unless they have been legally emancipated.

2. **You have been declared mentally incompetent by a physician to make your own decisions.** Incompetence might be due to a number of different reasons that would include dementia, developmental delays, and mental illness. For example, actively suicidal patients would not be allowed to refuse admission, nor would they be allowed to leave the hospital. In fact, suicidal patients — or any patient deemed to be a danger to themselves or others — can legally be held against their will for a 72-hour observation, or even longer with the involvement of a judge. There are also situations of what we'll call temporary incompetence. An example of this would be during a surgery, for example, where the surgeon finds he or she needs to perform more extensive surgery or a different surgery than was originally planned. The patient, since they are or have been under the influence of general anesthesia, would not

be considered competent to make the treatment decision until the anesthetic had been out of their system for 24 hours. In those cases, surgeons will approach the next of kin and discuss it with them. This is why it is so important to have a durable power of attorney for healthcare, which is discussed in the Legal Documents chapter.

3. **You have a current medical condition that is thought to impair your judgment.** For example, you're brought to the emergency room after a car accident. You have obvious and serious injuries; you are acting inappropriately and at the same time, you are refusing treatment. Emergency department physicians will assume that you are currently incompetent to refuse treatment because you may have a head injury. The hospital will treat you in a manner to which a competent person would have consented.

4. **You are under the obvious influence of alcohol or drugs that impair thinking and judgment.** Emergency room physicians are familiar with patients having a heart attack brought on by street drug use and who are not cooperative. Again, the physician will go ahead and treat the patient in a manner in which a competent patient would (based on the experience of other patients) want to be treated. How is this done? Doctors use sedatives to gain a patient's cooperation. When they sober up and are advised that they were uncooperative and had refused treatment, they usually don't remember refusing treatment and are grateful for the care.

Tips to Equip: Do you need a PPHA? What type is best for your needs?

A private professional healthcare advocate can:

1. **Understand complex medical situations** and advocate on you or your family's behalf with hospital administration in a way that is more likely to have your case not only heard, but resolved, in a manner that is best for the patient.

2. **Ensure that all your healthcare needs are met** in several ways. A medically trained PPHA can help clarify all your options and ensure that you have access to the essentials needed for a successful outcome.

3. **Protect you legally** (while making sure your wishes/ rights are respected), in many cases, better than attorneys. They are more familiar with medical jargon that has legal implications.

4. **Become your right-hand supporter and patient care manager,** whether by talking with insurance companies to get additional benefits, arranging for proper medical supplies and care providers, overseeing the quality of care given by home health aides and nurses, talking with your doctor, and arranging complex documentation necessary for cost-effective care. As many patients have told us: it's like having a nurse in the family!

Chapter 6

Emergency Care and Your Rights

What images come to your mind when you think of the emergency room? For the inexperienced, it might be George Clooney or Patrick Dempsey as a handsome doctor. For others, the thought of the ER elicits hand-wringing sweat and fear.

The first issue to consider: whether to call an ambulance. The decision to call is never taken lightly; most patients are worried about the cost. Another surprising concern many patients cite is that they don't want the neighbors to know what's going on when the ambulance pulls up outside the house. Here's some harsh reality, based upon the experience of emergency department physicians.

1. **In the event of any type of chest pain or breathing difficulty, an ambulance should always be called.** Emergency physicians cannot count the number of times they have had to meet a deceased patient and their completely traumatized family member/driver in a private car parked at the entrance of the ER. The family member usually says, "I wanted to call the ER, but he wouldn't let me." During a heart attack, a portion of the heart muscle itself is not receiving the blood (and therefore oxygen) that it requires, and the electrical wiring can be affected and trigger ventricular fibrillation. Medical people call this lethal rhythm "v-fib," and the only effective treatment for

it is defibrillation. It must be started within six minutes of the onset of this rhythm, or the patient's brain will suffer irreversible damage. If the heart attack victim is in a private car when this v-fib starts, there is *absolutely nothing* the driver can do to help the victim. Contrast this to the same heart attack victim being in an ambulance. An ambulance has a trained paramedic in the back of the rig with the patient, who is hooked up to the heart monitor. The moment that v-fib should begin, the paramedic can grab the defibrillator and, at that moment, has the best chance of shocking the patient's heart out of the lethal rhythm. Many successful "saves" have been made with the defibrillator readily available. Defibrillators are found in many public places now, and are simple enough for a second-grader to operate. Most airports, sports stations, schools, bus stations, malls, grocery stores, and many places of worship will have defibrillators on hand. It is best that the operator has taken a CPR course, but operating the defibrillator untrained is much better for the patient than doing nothing at all and waiting for paramedics to arrive.

2. **In the event of any stroke symptoms, an ambulance should always be called.** Think of a stroke as a heart attack in the brain. In most cases, a stroke is caused by a blood clot that disrupts the flow of blood (and oxygen) to the brain. In much fewer cases, a stroke is caused by a blood vessel that ruptures inside the brain, causing bleeding. The average layperson cannot tell the difference, and the action of a loved one will be the same: call 911. There are many different symptoms of strokes, but common ones include:

- Weakness on one side of the body, be it just an arm, just a leg, or both an arm and a leg
- Slurred speech, or not making any sense when you are speaking
- A drooping smile
- Passing out

Most people won't have all of these symptoms—or they may have completely different ones, depending upon the area of the brain affected. The best advice to give is that if you're not sure if it's a stroke, but things don't seem right, it is better to call the ambulance.

So why do you need an ambulance for a stroke? Many people falsely believe that nothing can be done for a stroke. These days, some hospitals (usually only major medical centers) can administer a medication called a clot-buster to break up a large stroke. This medicine does not come without serious risks, so it isn't used for minor strokes, but it may be tried on a major stroke involving a large part of the brain. To qualify to receive this clot-busting medication, you must receive the clot-buster medicine within three hours of your symptoms starting. If you wait a couple hours to see if the symptoms stop, you may very well be too late. By the time you drive to the hospital, get admitted to the ER, see the doctor, and get a CT scan, you may be outside of your three-hour window for treatment. If you call the ambulance at the onset of symptoms, you stand the best chance for treatment of a massive stroke.

In the event of any medical issue that appears to be an immediate threat to life or an arm or leg, an ambulance should always be called. "Better safe than sorry" is a good motto for medical emergencies.

If time permits, grab the important documents. This is especially true for someone who has chronic medical problems; who is in the middle of a complicated treatment, such as chemotherapy; or who has had several medical problems in the past. The documents should be kept together, ready to go in the event of a call to 911. You will receive faster and more skilled care with the presence of said documents. The ER physician won't spend time looking for your records; they will instead be spending time looking at you. These important documents include:

- **A list of all current medications**, their strength, when they are taken, what they're for (every empowered patient should have a general understanding of what each medication is for), and who prescribes it. This list should also include vitamins and herbal supplements, as some of them will interfere with or have a harmful interaction with medications that may be given at the hospital.

- **A list of all the physicians that you see**, along with their phone numbers.

- **A list of all allergies — medications and foods.** Along with the allergy, document what your allergic reaction is. Some unpleasant side effects of medication are called allergies by some patients; one example is penicillin. Many patients develop diarrhea when they take penicillin, and they will call this an allergy when it is really just an unpleasant side effect. The same goes for codeine; patients will get nauseated with codeine, and label it an allergy when, again, it is just an unpleasant side effect. Why does this matter? If you label yourself

106

allergic to penicillin when you aren't, you are limiting your physician's options for treating infections. If you mistakenly label yourself allergic to codeine, you are limiting your physician's options for treating your pain.

- **A list of past medical problems and past surgeries**; you can ask your physicians to each write up a list for you so you know it is accurate.

- **Your healthcare power of attorney** and your POLST (Physician Orders for Life-Sustaining Treatment) document, if you have either one. More on these in the Legal Documents chapter.

- **Copies of your insurance cards and driver's license** for ease of documentation.

In the event that you must call an ambulance, have someone stand outside and flag them down. Ambulances can have trouble finding addresses; this is a simple way to save time during an emergency.

The challenges that people face when they land in the emergency room can make equipping and empowerment extremely difficult. Most commonly, an ER visit is unexpected. Medical emergencies can be a sudden crisis or a worsening of a chronic condition. The physicians and nurses working there typically don't know the patient (though there are patients who are in the emergency room so often that ER staff will quietly refer to them as "frequent fliers"). It can be difficult to get your concerns conveyed because the staff is generally working at a fast pace to tend to multiple emergencies at one time. Some hospital emergency rooms might have upwards of 50-60 treatment beds with maybe three doctors working! To add to it, patients and their loved ones often don't have a clear understanding of the patient's medical conditions, medications, or their rights.

To know your rights, you must be informed about EMTALA, short for the Emergency Medical Treatment and Active Labor Act. When you present to the emergency room, you have the right to:

1. A medical screening exam to determine if an emergency condition exists.

2. Stabilization and treatment of emergencies, if possible.

3. Be transferred to a hospital that can treat you, if you cannot be stabilized in the facility where you initially present.

Confusing, right? Let's look at a few examples to clarify. Say you are a Medicare Advantage patient, meaning that specific doctors and hospitals are contracted to see you. You can't just show up anywhere you wish; it is essentially a Medicare HMO plan. You are across town visiting a friend when you fall and you have a pain in your hip. You are brought to an emergency room not on your health plan. Will they see you, even though they're not on your health plan?

Yes. You have a right to a medical screening exam to determine if a medical emergency condition exists. In this case, you would be screened to rule out a broken hip or other injuries from your fall. If indeed you had broken your hip and required surgery, you would then have the right to stabilization and treatment of your broken hip. Now, say that the hospital you landed in doesn't have an orthopedic surgeon on staff; you would then have the right to be transferred to a hospital that can treat you.

What about labor under EMTALA? If you are pregnant and in active labor, you are not going anywhere until that baby is delivered, unless the hospital doesn't offer obstetrical services.

Transferring a pregnant person in active labor is a big no-no!

Who can do what to help you in the ER?

In the olden days, the emergency room was just that—a room, staffed by inexperienced interns fresh out of medical school. There was little or nothing to be done for many medical emergencies because the technology had just not been developed. In 1979, the American Board of Emergency Medicine was created and emergency medicine became an official medical specialty, much like general surgeons or neurologists. Physicians trained in emergency medicine will staff most emergency departments, in all but the most isolated hospitals. In rural areas, where they may not be able to attract specialty physicians to the area, family practitioners or internal medicine specialists may still staff emergency rooms.

Today's emergency medicine specialists complete medical school, followed by a year of internship and three years of specialty training. They spend time in the emergency department and in various areas of the hospital, such as the operating room, obstetrics/gynecology, pediatrics, and the general medical floors to gain an understanding of all aspects of medicine. ER docs have to know a lot, but they can't know everything! They specialize in recognizing and treating medical emergencies, mass casualties, and disasters. They are definitely not there to replace your primary care physician.

An important note: when you come to the emergency room, the physicians there are only examining you for life-threatening emergencies. When Patient L shows up complaining of chronic back pain for six years, they likely will not receive an extensive amount of testing. The ER doctor will rule out *life-threatening causes* of back pain; if those aren't found, the doc will likely send the patient on their way to follow up with their primary care physician as an outpatient. That is not bad care on the part of the physician; it's just reality. The emergency room is only there to look for medical emergencies, plus routine visits to a PCP will help prevent emergencies in the first place.

Who's on duty at the emergency room?

1. **ED physicians.** ED stands for emergency department; it means the same as the emergency room. ED physicians are usually contracted by the hospital and are not typically hospital employees. What does this mean to you? You will receive a separate bill for their services, and in the case of allegations of medical malpractice, the hospital will quickly distinguish their liability from that of the ED physician.

2. **NPs or PAs.** A NP is a nurse practitioner—a registered nurse who has obtained additional training and certification to see patients on their own, with a physician co-signing their chart. A PA is a physician assistant, someone who has completed an undergraduate degree and two years of a graduate program designed to assist the physician in seeing patients. In some states, PA's can now see patients without a doctor co-signing; this was covered in a previous chapter. Be sure and ask about the training of the person who is treating you. Remember your patient's rights.

3. **RNs.** Registered nurses—we couldn't do without them.

4. **PCTs.** Patient care technicians (or "techs") do so much for patients these days and truly are the right hand of the registered nurses. They frequently put the patient in the

room, help them change into a gown, hook up monitors, and provide comfort. The only thing they can't do is administer medications; that is the job of the registered nurse.

5. **Scribe.** This is a person whose sole function is to take notes for the physician while they are speaking with you. They are a time-saver, and since they are only focused on taking notes, they can be more thorough. You may not even notice the scribe because they frequently stand in a back corner and don't ask any questions.

6. **EKG technician.** This individual has completed training in obtainment and general interpretation of the EKG (electrocardiogram). Don't be shocked if the EKG technician is a male, and you are a female patient and they ask you to expose your chest. It is their job. If you are uncomfortable, feel free to ask for a nurse to be present while the EKG is being obtained.

❖ **Respiratory therapist.** According to the Bureau of Labor (Bureau of Labor Statistics, 2015), respiratory therapists "[a]ssess, treat and care for patients with breathing disorders. Assume primary responsibility for all respiratory care modalities, including the supervision of respiratory therapy technicians. Initiate and conduct therapeutic procedures; maintain patient records; and select, assemble, check, and operate equipment." If you require specialized breathing care, you'll likely be meeting a respiratory therapist.

7. **Orthopedic technologist,** sometimes known as a cast technician. Their professional organization, The National Association of Orthopedic Technologists, says this

(National Association of Orthopedic Technologists, 2013): "The OT is able to fit and adjust canes, crutches and walkers, as well as giving patient instruction on the use of these walking aids. Other important responsibilities of the OT are the ability to apply simple braces, prosthetics, perform minor adjustments and repairs, as well as fabricate splints for various conditions under the direction of the orthopedic surgeon." Please do not confuse OT (orthopedic technologist) with an OT (occupational therapist); they are totally different fields!

Other hospital staff that you may find helpful during your visit:

1. **Charge nurse.** The emergency department charge nurse is in charge of the nurses during that particular shift. If you are having troubles with your nurse (or your physician, for that matter), it is wise to ask to speak to the charge nurse.

2. **Emergency department nurse manager.** This individual may or may not be working when you're in the emergency room. They are the manager of the ER. If you aren't getting anywhere with the charge nurse, the nurse manager is the next one up the chain.

3. **Hospital patient advocate.** Please do not confuse a private professional healthcare advocate with a hospital patient advocate! Hospital patient advocates are employees of the hospital. Their job is to serve the best interests of the hospital. When they interact with patients, they are there to help the hospital avoid getting sued. However, a hospital patient advocate can help with certain matters, like pain control. If you feel your pain is not being adequately addressed in the

ER, asking for the hospital patient advocate can help. For matters more medically complicated, you'll need a private professional advocate. Hospital patient advocates aren't going to look at every detail of your care; they are simply going to address the concerns that you voice. And they won't be able to spend unlimited amounts of time with you, either. Those roles would be left to a private advocate who only has your best interests at heart.

4. **Hospital social worker.** Social workers in hospitals are experts at nursing home placement, and are quite knowledgeable about Medicare and Medicaid regulations.

5. **Hospital pastoral care.** Enough cannot be said for pastoral care. These pastors will hold your hand through a crisis, pray with you, call family members, and sit with you during your most difficult times.

6. **Risk management department.** Their job is to address the hospital's legal matters. Whether it's avoiding a lawsuit, settling a lawsuit, or going to court, this is the department that handles it all. In some cases, private professional healthcare advocates contact the risk management department when things are going catastrophically wrong. While considered a dramatic and last-ditch step, it is incredible how much can change when risk management becomes involved. Could a patient contact the risk management department? Probably, but even simply asking for their phone number may get you the improvements in your care that you need.

Think of the dynamic ER environment like an elaborate ballet. Doctors and staff change in and out at shift change, or when going to lunch, or when going on break. Add to this a litany of patients:

some just arriving, some waiting to be seen, some in the middle of testing, some in the middle of treatment, some staying to be admitted, and some being discharged… all at the same time. If the ER is not managed well, it can feel exceptionally scary and chaotic to patients and their loved ones, and there can be many cracks in the system due to all of this constant change!

As you can imagine, the ER is unpredictable. One minute it's extremely quiet (though many people who work in the ER are superstitious and will never use the q-word for fear of an onslaught of patients), and the next moment there are multiple ambulances arriving with all sorts of emergencies, not to mention the horribly ill patients arriving via private transportation. Many times in the ER, patients are admitted but must wait on a hospital room, so they take up a room in the emergency department and continue to require care there until a room is available for them. If you find yourself amongst the "waiting for a room upstairs" category in the ER, feel free to ask for a hospital bed to be brought in. You'll be much more comfortable, and will rest just a bit easier. Always keep in mind your rights as a patient!

For the patient, one of the most important and potentially dangerous parts of the emergency department is the triage area. Think of triage registered nurses as the gatekeepers to the Magic Kingdom known as the emergency department. Typically, RNs are trained to work in triage. They are the ones who first perform an initial assessment of the severity of your condition — and here lies the potential for trouble.

The triage nurse decides upon the following: is your problem urgent? Do you need a room right now no matter what? Is your problem emergent, meaning that you get the next room that becomes available after the urgent folks are roomed? Or is your problem deemed non-emergent? If you are labeled non-emergent, it could be a very long wait for you in the ER, as you will be bumped down the queue for every urgent and emergent patient that arrives. Typical ER visits can last from four to eight hours, so I tell all my clients to go to immediate care clinics whenever possible for a much shorter wait time.

A 55-year-old woman was brought to a busy urban ER by her family because she was "acting crazy, not herself." The triage nurse performed their assessment on the patient, and deemed her non-emergent. Probably just another patient for the mental health department. The family, very respectful and polite, tried to calm her as she screamed uncontrollably and rolled around on the floor of the waiting room. They trusted that the triage nurse was correct in her assessment that this did not constitute a true emergency. By the time the security guards dragged this poor patient to a cart in the ER (she couldn't even walk at that point), it was quickly determined that she was suffering a massive heart attack. Her heart stopped and she could not be saved.

Her "crazy" behavior was likely a lack of oxygen circulating to her brain from the massive heart attack. The triage nurse made a judgment call, and in this case it was fatally inaccurate. What could've been done differently?

Had the family known their rights, they could have insisted that she be taken to the back and evaluated by a physician. There are too many stories of innocent errors in the triage area that have delayed patients' care, worsened their outcome, and/or even cost them their lives. We are all human and can all make mistakes; our job as empowered patients and families is to have the courage to buck the system and speak up when things don't go as planned.

Tips to Equip: Your rights during your emergency department visit

You have the right to:

1. **Have access to emergency services** (screening and stabilization) even if the hospital is out of your network and without financial penalty (remember EMTALA!).

2. **Take part in treatment decisions.** Just because you're a senior citizen or you are hard of hearing doesn't mean that you don't have a say in your own treatment.

3. **Ask about pros and cons of treatment (even no treatment).**

4. **Refuse any test or treatment** (if you are deemed competent as discussed in the Patient Bill of Rights Chapter).

5. **Discharge yourself from the hospital, even against medical advice.** However, if you sign yourself out AMA, your insurance company may stick you with the hospital bill.

6. **Respect and consideration.** Don't put up with surly nurses and rude physicians.

7. **Privacy of health information.** This should go without saying, right? No one should be yelling your weight across the room to the other nurse

8. **Complaints and appeals.** You have the right to complain, and you have the right to appeal without retribution.

9. **Ask for, remember (or write down), and use names of staff.** Everyone loves to hear their name being used in a positive tone, and people tend to treat you better when

they know that you know their name.

10. **If the patient isn't able to speak for themselves, or doesn't feel up to it, have one family member do the talking for the entire family.** It irks hospital staff to keep answering the same questions to different family members.

11. **Take notes** to recall what was said for review at a later time.

Tips to Equip: If your ER visit isn't going well

1. **Ask for your nurse** to come to the room and calmly discuss the issues. Remember, calm and rational win the fight. Anger and scare tactics will get you removed by hospital security.

2. If your nurse isn't helpful, **go up the chain.** Ask for the charge nurse. If they can't help, then ask for the emergency department nurse manager.

3. **Have the ER physician summoned to the bedside.** Ask direct questions in a calm and respectful tone. Avoid name-calling or threats to sue.

4. If all else fails, **ask for risk management's phone number** and call. Oftentimes, just asking for the number will bring about sweeping changes in your care.

Tips to Equip: The discharge process if you're in agreement

1. **Try to obtain copies of labs, X-rays, CT scans, EKGs, and any other test results to take with you.** It makes follow-up with your physician much easier and more streamlined.

2. **Ask the ED physician to phone your primary care doc before discharge to arrange follow-ups** if they haven't already done so. When an ED physician told Patient S to see a dermatologist in the next few days for her unexplained rash, she was shocked when she phoned the dermatologist and was told there was a six-month wait for an appointment! However, if a doctor phones another doctor and asks for that doctor to see you, you'll be seen the next day in most cases. If you call the same doctor on your own, chances are you'll be waiting for months.

3. **Make sure you understand discharge meds and instructions.** I cannot emphasize this enough. In fact, Medicare will enact a new law soon that requires hospitals to educate you and your family about how to take care of yourself at home. Right now, patient education in hospitals is woefully lacking!

Tips to Equip: *When you don't agree with discharge*

Without a doubt, this would be a great time to have a private professional healthcare advocate. But if you don't have access to one:

1. **Remain calm** and state your concerns to the physician.

2. **Take notes** as the physician gives you their reasoning. Seeing you take notes makes physicians think more thoroughly about their words and actions. It demonstrates your concern for what they are saying, and also serves as evidence if something goes wrong.

3. **Be firm in your convictions** if you still can't agree with the decision.

4. If the physician is still planning discharge, **go up the chain:** charge nurse, emergency department nurse manager, and then risk management.

Tips to Equip: Admission to the hospital from the emergency department

1. If there are no rooms available in the hospital, and it looks like a long wait in the ED, **request that a hospital bed be brought in**. You don't need to throw your back out sleeping on an ER cot when you're already ill with something else.

2. **Get clarification on drinking and eating restrictions.** It's amazing how many patients starve while in the ER waiting on a room, and then can easily get a meal when they get to their room.

3. **If on Medicare, ask whether you are on observation status or a full admission.** This is a complicated issue, and the ER physician may not have a say in this. If you are on observation status, you are considered an outpatient, and Medicare will not pay for your medications in the hospital. In addition, if you are admitted under observation status and you need to go to a rehab facility, you are going to be stuck with the rehab facility bill. You cannot, under current Medicare laws, go to rehab without first spending three midnights as an inpatient in a hospital. (More on this in the Medicare chapter.)

4. **If you are being admitted under observation status, ask if you can bring in your usual medications from home.**

   If they allow it, you can save a bundle of money on meds.

Chapter 7

Dangers Lurking In Every Hospital

In the past fifteen years, patient safety and medical error have been major areas of concern in hospitals throughout the country. In 2000, a landmark report was published that shook the medical establishment to its core: _To Err Is Human: Building a Safer Health System_ (Linda T. Kohn, 2000). The report was written by The National Academy of Sciences (NAS), a group that describes themselves as "a private, nonprofit society of distinguished scholars charged with providing independent, objective advice to the nation on matters related to science and technology."

One of the authors of the report, Linda T. Kohn, further describes the organization's mission: "Upon the authority of the charter granted to it by the Congress in 1863, the Academy has a mandate that requires it to advise the federal government on scientific and technical matters" (Linda T. Kohn, 2000). The scholars in the committee noted that as the healthcare system becomes more complex, more opportunities arise for medical error.

The NAS defined a few terms necessary to understand their findings:

1. **Safety:** freedom from accidental injury.

2. **Adverse event:** injuries caused by medical management. Some adverse events are preventable, such as an infection the patient acquires due to improper hand washing by the

medical staff.

3. **Error:** "the failure of a planned action to be completed as intended (i.e., error of execution), or the use of a wrong plan to achieve an aim (i.e., error of planning)" (Linda T. Kohn, 2000).

Through examining hospital admissions data from 1997, the report concluded the following:

1. Death caused by preventable adverse events occurred in at least 44,000 patients and possibly as many as 98,000 patients.

2. Medical errors are the eighth leading cause of death in the United States; that is more deaths than from motor vehicle accidents or breast cancer.

3. The NAS estimated the total national cost for preventable adverse events to be between $17 billion and $29 billion.

4. Medication errors account for one out of 131 outpatient deaths.

5. Medication errors account for one out of 854 inpatient deaths.

A 1997 study published in the medical journal Lancet reported, "In a study of 1,047 patients admitted to two intensive care units and one surgical ICU, 45.8 percent were identified as having had an adverse event, where adverse event was defined as "situations in which an inappropriate decision was made when, at the time, an appropriate alternative could have been chosen" (Andrews, Stocking, & Krizek, 1997).

In 2013, another study regarding medical error was published in the Journal of Patient Safety: "A New, Evidence-Based Estimate of Patient Harm Associated With Hospital Care" (John T. James, 2014). The author conducted a literature review of four previous medical error studies and found that the estimated 44,000 to 98,000 deaths per year due to medical errors noted in the *To Err Is Human* report was a low estimate. He concluded that between 210,000 and 400,000 patients per year died due to medical error in hospitals — unsurprising to those of us who work in hospitals. It's similar to any other industry; those who work within know exactly what happens behind the scenes.

John James, the author of the study, concluded with this statement regarding the goal of reducing deaths due to medical error: "Fully engaging patients and their advocates during hospital care, systematically seeking the patients' voice in identifying harms, transparent accountability for harm, and intentional correction of root causes of harm will be necessary to accomplish this goal." We couldn't agree more, and we believe that private professional healthcare advocates are the perfect way to reduce medical error and preventable deaths.

Personally? I believe these staggeringly horrible figures are still low. They are only the reported cases, and I know from observation within the medical system that there are wide variations in what happens versus what gets reported by the institutions themselves. Healthcare reimbursement for services is now very closely tied to a facility's safety statistics, and there is fierce competition to keep these numbers down. Hospital employees' salaries are often (at least indirectly) tied to their unit's rate of falls, infections, and medication errors.

About the incidence of medical error and the accuracy of reporting: you never know the real picture unless you work in a hospital setting every day. The problem is very real, and within each of us is hidden the best defensive tool available: our instincts. Every one of us knows what it feels like to sense when something is not right. Use your senses and instincts to alert you whenever you encounter a warning bell. That bell in our head is there to warn us of danger, and we should be alert and observant whenever we or our loved ones are hospitalized. If something doesn't seem right, speak up and voice your concerns to hospital staff. Don't be rushed into signing consent forms for procedures you don't understand.

Most people view hospitals as safe places: a respite when you are ill and need healing. They've got to be the cleanest place in town, right? You hear about "hospital corners" on beds (the best-made beds around) and "hospital clean."

We briefly discussed your right to expect a clean and safe environment in the previous chapter. Now we will further drill down to exactly what is safe and what is clean, as well as what you should expect when you receive care in a medical facility.

First off, the assumption that hospitals are extremely clean could not be further from the truth. Infections acquired while in the hospital are rampant and can be lethal. Why? The germs (usually bacteria) found in hospitals have been exposed to many powerful antibiotics. While most germs are killed by the antibiotics, a few of the germs that have been exposed to the multitude of antibiotics survive because they have figured out the game and genetically mutated, so that they are no longer killed by the antibiotics. These "superbugs" are known as antibiotic-resistant; they know how to survive antibiotics. Not only do they survive, they multiply.

There are now bacteria for which science has no cure. Hospital-acquired infections (HAIs) are on the rise.

An elderly patient had a worn-out hip joint that needed to be replaced. They were in reasonably good health, and were medically cleared for the surgery. The patient would have done extremely well — except that the new joint became infected, leaving them in a nursing home and on IV antibiotics for months. The new joint had to be surgically removed and replaced with another new joint, only to find out that the bacteria had colonized in the joint and can never be eradicated.

The United States Centers for Disease Control and Prevention (the CDC) reports that on "any given day, 1 in 25 hospitalized patients has at least one healthcare-associated infection."

The CDC divides HAIs into three categories:

1) Surgery and catheter-related infections.
2) Infections spread between patients.
3) Improper antibiotic usage.

Six common and often antibiotic-resistant bacteria cause many of these infections. Some bacteria, such as staphylococcus, live as a normal part of our skin, but when they enter a body cavity or an open wound, they cause an infection.

The culprit for the spread of many of these germs is very simple–the hands! Yes, the hands of the healthcare workers we entrust to restore our health. Improper hand cleansing is thought to be the culprit in many hospital-acquired infections.

Infection is an invasion of the body by germs. When you cut yourself at home, the cut may get a little red but you put some antibiotic ointment on it with a bandage, and it gets better. Germs at home tend to be very easy to control because they haven't been exposed to massive amounts of antibiotics. Unfortunately, the germs found inside hospitals are the strongest and deadliest known to mankind. Currently, there are bacteria for which there is no effective antibiotic, and they are found inside hospitals. How would those bacteria reach you? Hospital personnel, either on themselves or on their equipment, would bring it to you.

Patients and their advocates need to be extremely vigilant and not be afraid to speak up when they see activity that doesn't seem right. There is a massive grey area between clean and sterile. Clean is just what we think of: washed. In a clean environment, bacteria are still present, but hopefully the numbers are low and they are just the normal bacteria that live on the surface of our skin. Taking blood pressure would be a procedure where clean (as opposed to sterile) is all we need, since we are not breaking the surface of the skin. Gloves that come about 50 per box in a patient room are clean, but not sterile. They are fine for touching the outer surfaces of the skin, but not for procedures where skin will be broken. Sterile gloves can be identified by their being wrapped individually and double.

Medication errors and complications as a result are another significant risk in the hospital and outpatient setting. Becker's Hospital Review lists ten safety issues in hospitals, many of which patients cannot do much about (such as building maintenance and cyber security) but medication error was high on their list.

Deaths due to medication error are thought to account for one out of 894 hospital inpatient deaths and one out of 103 outpatient deaths (Linda T. Kohn, 2000). Medications can be lifesaving, but harmful if used in the wrong circumstance or given to the wrong patient. Nurses are trained to administer medication while following the "Six Rights" of medication administration: the right patient, the right medication, the right amount (dose), given by the right route (pill, IV, shot, or numerous others), the right time of day, supported by the right documentation.

Hospitals and pharmacies have policies and procedures in place to help reduce medication error, but accidents still happen. One major issue: vastly different medications that sound or look similar. The Institute for Safe Medicine Practices publishes an annual list formulated through medication and vaccine errors reported to them.

For medical personnel, the list is eye-opening. Imagine that you are given Xanax (a sedating, anti-anxiety drug) instead of Zantac (for heartburn). This medication "sound-alike" is just one example of hundreds! We have heard first hand of a patient who was supposed to get a TB test (PPD) and was mistakenly given a tetanus shot (Td) instead. What can you, as a patient or a loved one, do to help avoid these sometimes-deadly errors?

I got a call from a couple whose daughter had been transported to the emergency room after stopping a medication that managed her bipolar disorder. Their daughter was a professional, normally a very highly functional person, but bipolar patients sometimes think they do not need their medication when they are feeling well. When they stop their meds, life can get very interesting very quickly. In this case, the patient had left her husband and small children and gone to a hotel room with a heroin addict whom she was convinced was the love of her life. She drank herself into a near-unconscious state, and when her husband tracked her down, she threatened to kill herself. At that point, the patient was escorted to the local emergency room with the assistance of 911 and the EMTs.

She had been so violent that she needed to be put in restraints to keep her from doing harm to herself or others. Her alcohol level was over 300 (incredibly dangerous). After an hour or so she gave up fighting and convinced her nurses that she was fine, so her restraints were removed. She acted rational and eventually convinced her husband that he could leave to go outside for a smoke. I'm not sure what happened next, but when the nurses came back to her ER cubicle, she was frantically rummaging around the drawers in her area, having found partially used vials of controlled substances and shoved them into her pockets. I listened to their story with eyes wide open, thinking, "Really?" Unlocked narcotics and sedation in drawers in the emergency room are such a violation of hospital safety codes on so many levels that I was truly aghast. I worked in a critical care area for years and I know the hoops we have to go through to sign out, to waste [dispose of] and document controlled substances. I could not believe such a violation of patient safety had occurred.

The parents of this patient had contracted my services because the ER staff had called the police, who had her taken to a local psychiatric facility and promised they would prosecute her upon her release. I'm not saying that the patient had made good choices that night, but the fact was that she was drunk and high out of her mind, and her rights to safety were violated by leaving her unattended shortly after her arrival at the ER with a near-lethal alcohol level and threat of suicide. She simply could not be trusted, and the staff had a responsibility to have a sitter with her at all times. I'm sure they were horrified when they saw what she had found in the drawers, and calling the police seemed like the logical next step.

It was probably a good thing for the hospital that the parents called me instead of a lawyer, because that ER could have been shut down in a heartbeat. They might have even encountered a massive lawsuit on the grounds of a patient's safety being violated. I like hospitals and I have empathy for the ER staff's position, so I thought I'd take a softer tactic at first. I hate to see lawsuits against hospitals; the costs of multimillion-dollar lawsuits are, to me, one of the reasons why the cost of healthcare has skyrocketed over the years. I try to avoid lawyers at all costs. The day after I talked with the patient's parents, I made a friendly call to the hospital's risk manager. They have job security because every hospital in this country has their fair share of medical error; it's unavoidable, but it can be reduced.

I wanted her (the risk manager) to understand my role in this case. I very clearly understood that we had a major safety violation on our hands. My client's daughter was about to be arrested and likely lose her ability to work professionally due to the nature of her crime (she happened to be a nurse).

I said to the risk manager, "Help me understand what actually happened here, because I'm an ICU nurse and I know what we have to do to sign out and waste narcotics. I cannot imagine a suicidal, drunk patient being left alone in a room where there were unlocked narcotics. I'm sure there are pieces of the story that we're unaware of. Perhaps you'd like to go talk to the manager of the ER and find out what really happened. I'd like to see us avoid going to court over this, but the patient's parents are pretty upset about their daughter getting arrested when she leaves the psychiatric ward. The patient was blacked out and doesn't remember a thing. Do you think we can try to work this out?"

We got off the phone on a respectful note and I waited for a return call, which came about 45 minutes later. The charges against the patient were dropped without incident. Her parents made certain she received psychiatric follow-up, and calamity was avoided on the part of both parties. In this case, the patient's safety was compromised not only by her state of mind and mental health, but also by the staff's negligence in maintaining proper protocol. My advocacy for the patient's ultimate safety (career, reputation, health) once her health was restored resulted in a positive outcome for all parties involved.

Tips to Equip: The difference between clean and sterile

1. **Clean is not good enough when we go deeper than the outer surface of the skin. Sterile procedure should be practiced when dealing with surgical sites, IV sites, drawing blood, and taking care of wounds.** Sterile means free of living organisms. If a nurse tells you that she "can't draw blood wearing gloves," then ask for another nurse to draw the blood.

2. **Taking blood pressure is a "clean" activity, not a sterile one; we are not going below the skin surface.** Staff should be wiping their stethoscope head with alcohol before it touches your skin.

3. **Just wearing gloves is not enough.** All staff should either wash their hands with soap and warm water or use hand sanitizer when they enter your room, before touching you, and before donning gloves. They should also wash or use sanitizer as they leave your room. Gloves can have microscopic holes, allowing bacteria from another patient to colonize on you. The skin underneath needs to be clean.

4. **To wash your wound, staff should use sterile gauze as the "washcloth" to cleanse your skin.**

5. **Healthcare workers ideally should not be wearing acrylic nails;** all sorts of horrible bacteria are found underneath acrylic nails, and they cannot be scrubbed away. The CDC recommends that workers not wear acrylic nails when dealing with high-risk patients. The problem is that the CDC does not define a high-risk patient, but we personally feel that all hospitalized patients are at risk and acrylic nails should be avoided in all circumstances.

6. **The CDC recommends that healthcare workers with natural nails keep them trimmed to ¼ inch in length,** to reduce the numbers of bacteria under the nails (Centers for Disease Control and Prevention, 2016).

Tips to Equip: Avoid hospital-acquired infections

1. **Keep your hands clean in the hospital.** Here is a list from the CDC of when patients should wash their own hands:

   - Before preparing or eating food
   - Before touching your eyes, nose, or mouth
   - Before and after changing wound dressings or bandages
   - After using the restroom
   - After blowing your nose, coughing, or sneezing
   - After touching hospital surfaces such as bed rails, bedside tables, doorknobs, remote controls, or the phone

2. **If using alcohol-based sanitizer, your healthcare worker should put the product on their hands, make sure all surfaces are covered, and rub their hands together until they're dry.** This process should take around 20 seconds.

3. If the healthcare worker is washing using soap and water, they should first wet their hands, apply a hospital-approved soap, lather for at least 15 seconds while covering all surfaces of fingers and hands, rinse, dry hands with paper towel and use the paper towel to turn off the faucet.

4. The CDC has coined the phrase "speaking up for clean hands" and offers these tips:

   - **Ask your visitors to wash their hands.** When they first arrive, ask them to wash; after they've been there for a while, ask them to wash their hands again. (Think about them touching the furniture in your room, touching you, rides in the elevator, trips to the cafeteria and gift shop as sources of bacteria in a hospital!)

   - **Make sure to keep your own hands washed.**

   - **Don't be afraid to ask your healthcare worker to wash their hands again** if you didn't see them doing it. A clean environment is your right!

   - The CDC has a great line for talking to your healthcare workers about hand washing before performing any procedure. You can simply say, **"I'm worried about germs spreading in the hospital. Will you please clean your hands once more before you start my treatment?"** (Centers for Disease Control and Prevention, 2016)

5. **Urinary catheter infections are another common source of healthcare associated infections.** While appropriate right after surgery, or if you're too ill to get out of bed to use the bathroom, each day that a catheter is left in increases your risk of infection. Ask your physician each day, **"Do I still**

131

need this urine catheter?"

6. The same goes for your IV. Intravenous catheters are sitting in your vein, creating a direct pipeline for bacteria to travel from your skin into your bloodstream. Ask your physician each day, **"Do I still need this IV?"** The worst they can say is, "Yes, you still need it." If your IV is starting to look red, or is getting sore, please do speak up; it could mean that it's becoming infected.

7. **If you're going to have surgery, ask your surgeon how they prevent infections during their procedures.**

Tips to Equip: Avoiding medication errors

1. **Don't distract your nurse with idle conversation** when they are preparing to give you your medications, while they are discussing your medications with you, or while preparing for you to swallow them.

2. **Know your pills, in every way possible.** Know their names, the reason you take them, their strength (frequently this is in milligrams for pills), and the quantity of pills that you take in total. A caveat regarding recognizing your pills by sight is that you can't always go by a pill's appearance. Most facilities are using generic medications whenever possible now, and different manufacturers of the same medicine will produce pills of different shapes and colors than what you are accustomed.

3. **Have the nurse review every single pill with you before you swallow it.** The nurse administers your meds off of a medication order sheet, which is a personalized list of your meds and all their specifics. Follow along with the nurse as

they refer to your medication order sheet and prepare to pass you your medications. Have them recite the name, the strength, the purpose of the medication, and for what time of day it is ordered. The pills should be in their original packaging and should be shown to you in that packaging, so that you are certain that you are receiving the correct ones.

Many people will read these recommendations and think that this is way beyond the scope of being a patient. It probably is, but won't you rest easier knowing that you are receiving the correct medications ordered for you? This is called advocating for *yourself*. If the thought of doing all this double-checking causes you to have flashbacks to high school chemistry lab or the head-spinning days of algebra, then by all means consider hiring a private professional healthcare advocate (PPHA) to help oversee your care in the hospital. PPHAs with a nurse's or doctor's background have the education and experience to help prevent medical error and improve communication for hospitalized patients.

Tips to Equip: Protecting your safety while in the hospital

1. **Leave jewelry and other valuables at home.** For things that have been brought, there should be a way to lock your valuables so you are not a victim of theft.

2. **Report any unusual behavior by your roommate** (if you have one) or their visitors.

3. **Alert staff to any spills you see on the floor.**

4. Sometimes, hospitals need to keep patients safe from themselves. **Patients who are at risk of harming themselves or others should be provided a 24/7 sitter to stay in their**

room and make sure they're safe. It is the hospital's responsibility to provide a sitter at their own expense if the patient's safety is at risk. A few common scenarios:

- When left alone, suicidal patients could seek out medications and/or objects left behind in exam rooms and harm themselves.

- Patients with Alzheimer's or other forms of dementia can get confused in the hospital, fall out of bed, and suffer broken hips and head injuries.

- Patients intoxicated by drugs or alcohol in the emergency room need to be continually observed so that they do not wander out of the hospital and get hit by a car in the parking lot, or fall out of bed and hurt themselves or others; they are not in their right mind and their actions are unpredictable. It is the hospital's responsibility to keep them safe while they are under their care.

- Weak and confused elderly patients are often unaware of their limitations when they are ill, and medications will also make them more unsteady on their feet. If you notice an elderly person behaving in an unsafe manner while in the hospital, please alert the staff immediately. If you notice that your family member appears weak, confused or dizzy when standing, or they try to get out of bed on their own, please alert the staff to institute a fall risk protocol, so that they are more closely watched. If a patient is very confused, a family member may want to act as a sitter to watch their loved one at all times. If that is not possible, the hospital may provide a sitter to watch the patient at all times. Tell staff that you are concerned for their safety, and they will have to do something to provide for an extra layer of protection. You know your family member better than anyone, after all!

Chapter 8

Seniors: A High-Risk Group of Hospital Patients

I might refer to this chapter as my favorite within the book, as the elderly hold a special place in my heart. We see a lot of lonely seniors in our practice, and I continue to grow increasingly concerned for their safety. They worry me the most, especially those with no family available to help them ask the right questions, tell their history, or provide the correct list of medications and allergies when they need help. Unfortunately, this population is growing, day-by-day, in our society as baby boomers age, spouses die, children live on the other side of the country, and physical challenges grow every year.

Some call them "senior orphans" or "solo-agers," but at the very least, they are vulnerable in today's fast-paced healthcare landscape. These seniors (and adults with disabilities!) need a friend at their side to help them navigate the short-term as well as the long-term crises they encounter. If they have children who don't live nearby, oftentimes the children do not even realize how much their parents are struggling when they only get in contact once or twice a year.

One of our recent clients had a typical hospital experience. His family had contacted us several months prior from out of state when they grew alarmed about the poor quality of care he was receiving in a nursing home. A series of unfortunate medical events had resulted in kidney failure, weakness, weight loss, and multiple facility-acquired infections. He was only 73 years old and he looked 85. Within a day, we transferred him to a good hospital, where his infections were treated and he was discharged to a high-quality rehab facility with excellent physical therapy and low infection rates.

He was well on the road to recovery when he developed a urinary tract infection and needed to be re-hospitalized at a different hospital. He was weak, didn't feel well, and quickly developed confusion from sleep deprivation, a bed sore from lying motionless all the time, severe malnutrition, and another infection. Nobody got him out of bed to a chair or helped him eat, and he grew weaker every day. His nurse advocate addressed his concerns daily with staff, but he continued to decline — and then the weekend came around, and most follow-through ground to a halt.

Five days into the hospitalization, the staff started telling his niece that he should probably go into hospice. Because of hospital neglect? Not on my watch!

I quickly informed them that the patient himself did *not* want to give up now. No one had even discussed hospice with him. I suggested that they needed to call in a gastroenterologist and start feeding him quickly. (A consult submitted three days prior had never been initialed.) We canceled the hospice consult, spent hours at the hospital every day talking with all the doctors, and insisted upon more aggressive medical care.

He is back at rehab now and is slowly improving. Sadly, every day lying around in bed in the hospital translates into about a week of rehab post-hospitalization to get back to normal. He had five nurses in five days, so none of the nurses even knew what normal looked like for our client. Nurses mean well, but big-picture items are often neglected today due to the fast-paced hospital environment. The computer takes up so much time that nurses can often miss the forest for the trees. A patient refuses to get up? Fine. She can move on to the next task, the next patient. In the old days, it was considered standard nursing practice to make certain our patients got up and walked, ate, and did deep breathing exercises every shift to *prevent* a future rehab stay! Sadly, the core component of good nursing practice is being lost: patient advocacy.

The new breed of nursing graduates may be good at computerized charting, but critical thinking and common sense are lacking in many cases. Up to 25 percent of nursing school graduates are leaving the profession after two years, disillusioned victims of culture shock. A serious shortage of doctors and nurses is projected to be coming soon, and I understand why.

The elderly are particularly vulnerable to medical error when they enter the hospital. This again, speaks to the importance of routinely seeing a primary care physician. Part of the reason is because when they feel poorly, they don't eat. Physical therapy is not initiated early enough. They get weak easily and are sensitive to new medications that may cause confusion, falls, complications of bed rest, and hospital-acquired infections. Their immune systems are weaker to begin with, and they catch infections easily when they are around more germs.

We see so many unsuspecting cases of someone's mother going into the hospital for a pelvic fracture that leads to pain, which then leads to immobility and poor appetite. The downward spiral is inevitable as the immobility often leads to bed sores, pneumonia, and sleep deprivation. The sleep deprivation leads to confusion, which leads to falls and, ultimately, fractures. It is heartbreaking for families who have an implicit trust that, when they send grandma to the hospital for healing, the hospitalization actually results in further harm done.

At some point, the family may have to decide whether or not their parents are safe to continue living independently. That conversation alone can stir up a mixed bag of emotions; there are many things to consider. Will the parents come and live with their children? Are they safe to live alone? Is assisted living an option? What about their financial situation? Do they need a caregiver?

This is where a PPHA can become an invaluable asset, not only to the person who needs the care, but to provide an immense sense of relief to the family (who most likely are part of the Sandwich Generation we discussed earlier). They have no idea how to navigate this new world of taking care of mom and/or dad as well as their children and spouse, while possibly living half a country away from the parents.

It's a lot to consider. I hope the information presented here provides you with peace of mind, along with the tools you need to make informed decisions that are best for your unique situation.

Finding a primary care physician is more complicated than it used to be. Gone are the Marcus Welby medical care scenarios of the past, where it was just fine to have one family doctor who knew your history by heart. You could also count on seeing his familiar face wherever you needed to be seen: office, home, hospital, or ER.

Many patients wonder whether they should look for a family practice physician or an internal medicine physician. Knowing the difference between the two can help you decide. A family medicine physician is a doctor who has undergone a three-year family medicine residency, learning how to treat everyone from newborns to the elderly. In theory, a family medicine physician sounds good. They can steer the boat, if you will. They can become familiar with your entire family; you will see the same physician as your children and your spouse. They will get to know your family history, and that can possibly aid in their treatment of you. However, the practical problem is that depending on your needs, there is no realistic way any one physician can learn detailed care of every age group in just three years. But if you enjoy fairly good health, or if you want to be able to see the same doctor as your children, then a family medicine physician can be a great choice.

If your health needs are more complex (either due to a chronic, complex illness or aging), you may want to consider an internal medicine specialist. Internal medicine specialists are never trained in treating children, so they are considered a physician for adults. They spend three years in residency learning only adult care. Many medical specialists, such as geriatricians, hematologist/oncologists, cardiologists, and pulmonologists, first complete an internal medicine training, so it is the basis for a great deal of adult medicine. Geriatricians are generally trained in internal medicine, but their expertise and passion is focused on the care of older adults and healing common medical conditions in the elderly.

Finding a Good Physician

Many people ask us how to find a good physician. The truth is: it can be tricky. Internet sites like healthgrades.com or zocdoc.com are fine to search for the basics. You will usually be able to find the physician's contact information, educational background, board certifications, and possibly malpractice and sanction history at these sites. You will frequently find patient reviews there as well. Keep in mind, however, that physician recommendations are not always accurate. Disgruntled patients sometimes make completely false accusations, and some sites may have dozens of glowing recommendations posted by the office's marketing department.

Try to get a recommendation from a nurse or a doctor. Ask them to whom they would send their own family members. That is usually a pretty good endorsement. If you happen to find a physician on the internet, or a friend tells you about their physician, ask a nurse that you know (be sure you make it clear that this conversation is confidential — between you and them) which internist or family medicine specialist on staff at that hospital they would choose for their family to see. You probably won't get far if you word the question in other ways ("What do you think of Doctor V?"). Asking whom they would bring their family member to see will yield an honest and positive response, and you're not asking the nurse to say anything bad about any physician. You can do something similar if searching for a specialist: call the hospital's physician referral hotline and ask which physician they would recommend to a family member. Then do your homework. I have found that if doctors I know who work in hospitals will tell me who they send their own family members to, that is the best compliment of all.

Too many medications aren't necessarily a good thing!

We had a client whose son contacted us because his mother was becoming increasingly forgetful and dizzy at home. Upon review of her medications, we saw that she had been prescribed a sleeping pill that has dangerous side effects, particularly in elderly women. When she told her doctor that she was having problems during the daytime with restlessness and dizziness, he prescribed a second medication for anxiety that compounded her problems. Her doctor suggested that she might be developing Alzheimer's when, in fact, she was being overmedicated. Once she got a new doctor and was weaned off the medications, her symptoms disappeared and her son exclaimed, "I have my mother back again!"

Fortunately, this frail, elderly woman did not have any falls or accidents related to the dizziness she experienced as a result of her two psychotropic medications, but many seniors do have tragic consequences of being overmedicated. Unfortunately, patients often expect to receive a prescription for any problems they are experiencing when they go to a doctor. It is wise to remember that all medications have side effects, and the more one is on, the higher the risk of interactions that may lead to harm, injury, or even worse. This is particularly true for the elderly!

We recently got a call about a 92-year-old woman whose son was concerned about his mother's safety after she had sustained a fall, breaking three ribs. When we met her, we saw that this tiny woman was on 14 medications, five of which had side effects of vertigo. Older adults are more sensitive to medications, so they usually require lower doses than someone younger. One of the medications she was on was a powerful diuretic at a dose that a 40-year-old man would take. We were able to go to our client's doctor appointment with her the following week, which resulted in several medications being discontinued or lowered. Once the doctor saw on paper how many pills our client was taking, it was easy to see how many of them could cause the dizziness that had led to her fall. Some of them had also likely contributed to a gradual weight loss over the past six months as well. To support her continued and optimal health, a nutritionist that we now work with has been able to put her on a high-nutrition diet that her caregivers will help her follow. Even though our client is 92 years of age, her vision of quality of life includes living in her own apartment with the right support, and we are helping her do that.

Tips to Equip: Before you make your first appointment with a new doctor, ask:

1. Will I see the same person for primary care each time I come to the office?

2. What happens when I go to the hospital? (Will my primary care physician see me, or will I be assigned a hospitalist?)

3. Does the doctor accept Medicare and/or my insurance?

4. How long does it typically take to get an appointment if I am sick?

5. Can you tell me if the doctor has experience treating (my specific ailment)?

6. What hospitals does the doctor have admitting privileges at?

7. What is the office appointment cancellation policy?

8. Is there a policy for phone calls after hours? (Some offices will charge for after-hours phone calls.)

When you have an appointment with your new physician, it is best if you can bring a list of your current medications (prescription and over-the-counter), supplements, and vitamins that you're taking. Don't forget to write down any medications and/or foods that you're allergic to (some vaccinations, for example, are egg-based, so food allergies can still be important). Inform your new medical team of any past medical problems you've had, past surgeries, and current problems. Be up-front about other physicians that you're still seeing as well. It is important for physicians to communicate with each other. Having the information written down before you arrive is valuable, as it is easy to forget things when you're nervous.

Plan to arrive to your appointment about 15 minutes early to relax a bit (makes for better blood pressure readings) and fill out new patient forms. Be sure to introduce yourself to the staff, and try and learn their names too. It is helpful when you have to communicate over the phone with them in the future; it also helps them have a sense of who you are.

We discussed many of the following in the Patient Bill of Rights chapter, but your rights come into play from the very beginning of the doctor-patient relationship, not just when there might be a problem. When you meet a new physician, try and stay aware of how you're feeling about them. Are they making eye contact? Are they listening to my concerns, or cutting me off as I'm speaking? Do they seem rushed? Are my questions being answered to my satisfaction? Are my rights as a patient being respected? Am I being treated with respect and consideration? Do I have a role in discussing treatment options? If I disagree, am I being treated with respect? Is the physician more focused on the computer than on me as a person?

Medications: The Good, the Bad and the Ugly

Very few will argue that medications have the potential to prevent, modify, and cure disease as well as improve the length and quality of life. But are there downsides to these medications? To quote an old Western movie title, we need to consider the good, the bad and the ugly when contemplating whether to take a medication.

We've already discussed medication errors in the previous chapter. Let's examine some recent news reports regarding a very commonly used class of heartburn/gastroesophageal reflux disease (GERD) medications that physicians refer to as proton pump inhibitors (PPIs). We mere mortals know these meds by common brand names such as Nexium, Prilosec, and Prevacid, or generics such as omeprazole or esomeprazole, in addition to the plethora of other names used to reference them.

Here's the *good*: PPIs are extremely effective for heartburn/ acid reflux. They have improved the quality of life and prevented, as well as cured, serious gastrointestinal health problems for many, many people. Over the years, they have also been thought of as safe, so they are widely used. Their effectiveness and popularity are demonstrated by the many different PPIs available, both by prescription and over the counter.

Now here's the *bad* part: A recent medical study published in the Journal of the American Medical Association (JAMA) found an association between the use of PPIs and chronic kidney disease. Another recent study, published in JAMA Neurology, reports a statistical association between the use of PPI medications with a 1.4-fold increased risk for the development of dementia. We do need to make one thing clear here, and that is that an "association" does *not* prove that proton pump inhibitors *cause* dementia or chronic kidney disease; there is only a statistical association between their use and an increased risk for the development of these diseases. The reason for these associations is not understood, and to study cause-and-effect, randomized clinical trials will need to be performed. So while it's best to pay attention to news reports regarding medications, you need to keep in mind the potential problems and limitations of medical research and keep an open dialogue going with your physician regarding your medications.

Here's the *really ugly* part: untreated medical conditions can lead to other, more serious health problems, disability and early death. Much worse than the possible negative effects of a medication. So, leaving conditions untreated is most often not a good option. Even heartburn or GERD can have serious complications, and there is no disputing that PPIs have improved quality of life as well as treated serious health problems and saved many people's lives. While there are alternative treatments available for GERD, they may not be right for your unique circumstances, and you should not abruptly stop your PPI (or any other prescribed medication, for that matter) without first consulting your physician. Your body needs acid to break down protein in digestion, and PPIs are ideally meant for short-term use only.

But what of the rising costs of pharmaceuticals? Consumers are paying more for their medications, and they are not happy about it. To understand the "why" of any price increases in healthcare today, one has to understand the national impact that the Affordable Care Act has had on providers, insurers and pharmaceutical companies. To be simplistic, think of a balance scale or a seesaw on a playground. When reimbursement rates by Medicare or private insurers decrease, prices have to come up to balance out the bottom line. Pharmaceutical companies are using many strategies today to preserve their profit margin; and consumers are paying more out-of-pocket costs for most healthcare-related expenses, including prescriptions. Insurance companies are doing the same so they can remain profitable.

"Polypharmacy" is a new term for something many people already know far too well. Among seniors today, 44 percent of men and 57 percent of women over 65 take five or more medications every week. Twelve percent of seniors take over 10 medications weekly (American Geriatric Society).

When people take too many medications, often prescribed by different healthcare practitioners who do not communicate with each other, dangerous side effects and interactions can occur and go unnoticed until a crisis happens. It is important to always keep a complete list of medications with you at all times, so that all healthcare providers have correct information should you suddenly land in the hospital.

Taking medications is even more serious for older adults. As we age, our kidneys and liver do not break down medications as well, and a "normal" dose can quickly become toxic. Other times, medications just don't work well, or they give older people terrible side effects and leave them sicker than before they took the drug.

In 2012, the American Geriatric Society updated their Beers Criteria for Potentially Inappropriate Medication Use in Older Adults. This is an important document for seniors, as it lists medications that should potentially be avoided in older adults due to extreme side effects or increased risks of complications.

Many of the medications that made it onto the Beers Criteria list for use in older adults cause symptoms such as confusion, hallucinations, sleepiness, blurred vision, difficulty urinating, dry mouth, and constipation.

As you can imagine, if an older adult takes a medicine that makes them dizzy, they risk falling and breaking a hip or hitting their head, or having huge changes in their thinking abilities due to certain medications. Family members might believe their loved one is developing Alzheimer's disease when in reality, the changes in thinking they're seeing may just be due to medications.

If you have access to a computer, go to www.americangeriatrics.org and search Beers Criteria and you can view the medication list for yourself.

Tips to Equip: When your doctor gives you new medication, ask about:

1. **The reason they are recommending this medication.**

2. **The side effects** (side effects are bothersome things that may occur with a medication; usually not life threatening, but annoying. For example, drowsiness with Benadryl, or diarrhea with antibiotics).

3. **The dangers to taking this medication** (physicians refer to these dangers as adverse effects).

4. **Possible interaction with other medications.**

5. **Alternatives to taking this particular medication.**

6. **What could happen if this condition is not treated with medication.**

Tips to Equip: Questions to ask regularly about your medications

1. Do I still need this medication?

2. Have there been any reports I need to know about regarding the safety or effectiveness of this medication?

3. Are there any lifestyle modifications I can make to reduce or eliminate my reliance on this medication?

Tips to Equip: Keeping prescription costs down

1. **Always request a generic equivalent if your physician agrees** (there are a few brand-name medications that are clearly superior to generic, but for the most part, a medication is a chemical component that is the same no matter what the fancy name or packaging).

2. **While you are in the doctor's office getting that new prescription, ask for samples.** (Pharmaceutical reps give away billions of dollars' worth of meds a year to doctors at their offices in an effort to convince them of the superiority of their drug. Most of the time doctors forget about this option, so they have closets full of samples which will go to waste if they are not given away.)

3. Once you know you will be on the medication long-term, **request a 90-day prescription with three refills so you can get it from a mail-order pharmacy at deeply discounted costs.**

4. Finally, **don't forget to take advantage of drug discount cards** and do cost comparison on sites like **goodrx.com, WeRx.org,** and **LowestMed.com. NeedyMeds.org** has a huge

database of medications that may be subsidized for low-income people or those without insurance.

5. If you want to purchase your prescriptions online, **make certain any online pharmacy has the VIPPS (Verified Internet Pharmacy Practice Sites) seal on the website to make sure you avoid Internet scams.**

Tips to Equip: Managing the side effects of medications

1. **Keep a list of all of your prescriptions, over-the-counter medications, vitamins, and supplements that you take, along with their strength and how often you take them.** Bring this list to every physician at every appointment.

2. **Ask your doctor if any of your medications are known to have side effects.** Check the American Geriatric Society's Beers Criteria, and if any of your medications are on the list, ask your physician about whether that drug is right for you. To quote the American Geriatric Society, "Keep in mind that if a drug you take is on one of the lists in the *AGS Beers Criteria*, this does not necessarily mean that it poses greater risks than benefits *for you*. The way *you* respond to a medication or medications can differ from the way other people respond to it. This is why the experts who updated the criteria use the phrase *"potentially* inappropriate." While the drugs on the lists *may* cause side effects in some older adults, they won't necessarily cause these problems in *all* older people."

   • **Never discontinue taking a medication on your own without consulting your doctor.** Discontinuing some medicines suddenly can cause death or serious complications. An empowered, educated, and equipped patient is a smart patient who doesn't try to practice medicine without a license!

Chapter 9

Senior Orphans and Elder Abuse

What is a senior orphan? Simply put: it is a person over 65 who falls into one of three categories: (1) no family left; (2) family who has no regular contact with the isolated senior (i.e. dysfunctional families or those who live in other parts of the country); or (3) family who is taking advantage of the senior financially, depleting funds that may be needed for long-term care.

There is a growing concern among some of us who work in the senior care industry with the issue of elder financial abuse. Not only are seniors being taken advantage of by scam artists and "helpful" neighbors who weave their way into the vulnerable person's life and gain access to bank accounts and retirement funds, but I have noticed that many times, the perpetrator is most often a family member.

We regularly encounter sons and daughters who are reticent to approve needed expenses for their parents' long-term care because they are experiencing financial stresses themselves. They are afraid that there will be no inheritance left for them if Mom or Dad gets transferred to an assisted living facility or a high-quality skilled nursing facility. The reality is that higher-quality nursing homes rarely admit people when their resources are almost depleted and they are in the process of applying for Medicaid. The better skilled nursing facilities require at least one year of private pay from patients before they transition to Medicaid payments for skilled care.

Elder abuse can also be as simple as giving grandchildren a car when they are also living on limited means. Seniors love their grandchildren and want to see them enjoy gifts prior to their passing. When family members receive financial "gifts" from their parents or grandparents in the latter part of their lives, it may actually disqualify the senior from receiving Medicaid if they run through their savings and need to receive Medicaid benefits for long-term care expenses (more about this in the *Intricacies of Medicare* chapter). They justify the gift by telling themselves that the "black sheep" grandchild just needs a bit of help to get back on their feet and they anticipate dying before long anyway, so they just give it away now, so they can enjoy giving.

Running out of money before they die also happens to be one of the biggest fears faced by the aging population—even more so if they have no family to depend on. The good news is that there is help available. A wise financial planner and elder law or estate-planning attorney can often alleviate those fears, help seniors protect their assets, and avoid costly financial errors. There are many new and creative ways to help people protect their assets and plan wisely for long-term care needs. They can also help by offering solutions for what happens if they should run out of money and still look forward to many years of life to live and healthcare to receive.

The important thing to remember is that there are options, and no one needs to worry about being put on the street once their money runs out. This is also an important reason to find a "driver" to help your family navigate the course wisely. The fear of the unknown can be paralyzing, but I promise you this: it is always better to know your options rather than remain in the dark and suffer needlessly out of worry.

Earlier this year, I received a call from an attorney in another state who referred a woman to me that was reporting that she was being held in a nursing home against her will, and bad things were happening to her every day. To be honest, I first suspected that the woman may have had dementia or a mental illness, but I decided to go check it out myself—just in case—and report back to the attorney on my findings.

When I went to the nursing home, the front desk personnel were very friendly, and the main floor looked older, but fairly clean, so I took the elevator upstairs and walked into a crowded nursing station area. Flanked on one side of the hall, there were several pathetic-looking seniors tied into wheelchairs, crying and yelling, wailing and begging for help, while staff members stood by socializing in the nurses' station. They ignored the patients, who were obviously in advanced stages of dementia or perhaps even mentally unwell. I proceeded to the patient in question's room, anxious to see what I might find there.

Caroline, a petite woman of 76, sat in her bed waiting for me, and had a mask over her face and mouth. She was one of four patients in the room, and had been transferred to a four-bed ward after her 100 days of Medicare had run out. The other patients in the room wore blank stares, either curled up in a corner, trembling, or leaning over the side of the wheelchair they were strapped into. Caroline seemed anxious and began to tell me her story.

Thirty years ago, her husband left her and her four young children, divorcing her for a new woman he had met. He offered little support after the divorce, though he was a well-off businessman. He was foreign-born and she had met him when she traveled to the Middle East. His ethnic background was very patriarchal—women had few rights and were not respected as Americans generally have come to expect. Caroline was a traditional American, who had been raised to be independent. She refused to dwell on her unfortunate circumstances, but rather made the best of things and moved on. She put herself through school and earned a real estate license. She also started a home design and real estate company, and her children enjoyed the advantage of higher education. All four children were successful in their various careers.

Both the father and oldest son were reported to be alcoholics and philanderers, and as her children grew up, they gravitated more toward their father. They rarely visited their mother, and she was heartbroken. The oldest son and his wife lived in Canada and had a two-year old son, whom Caroline had not yet seen. When I met Caroline, she had been in three low-rent-type nursing homes in the past six months. She had one broken, dislocated wrist that had needed surgery for several months. She had not seen a doctor since arriving at the present nursing home two months earlier. Doctor appointments, MRI scans, and medicines had been canceled at the last moment on multiple occasions. She could not sleep for the loud wailing and crying of other patients in the halls every night. She often missed meals, or they arrived late and cold. The nurses gave her incorrect medications every day, or refused to give her meds that she had relied on for years to prevent recurrence of cancer that she had successfully been treated. She was distraught and desperate to leave the nursing home and return home with 24-hour caregivers, which she could afford since she owned several large properties in a prestigious suburb of Indiana.

When I asked her how she had come to be a nursing home patient, her story grew even more troubling. She suffered from several chronic medical conditions, and six months earlier she had gone to the hospital to undergo a CAT scan. Although she had told the tech that she was allergic to the dye used and the sedative they wanted to give her, they gave it to her anyway and she suffered an anaphylactic reaction, resulting in a cardiopulmonary arrest. She was put on life support, transferred to a major medical center, and woke up a week later. While she was incapacitated (even though she had named her oldest son her healthcare power of attorney years earlier) she found out that her son had hired a shark of an attorney to file a motion for an emergency guardianship order. This effectively took away all her rights to manage her own affairs or even pay her own bills. Her assets were frozen and her mortgage, taxes, licenses, and utilities were all unpaid and she was in danger of losing her properties.

At this point, I could not even contract with this client since she essentially had no legal rights, and was prevented by the court from even having access to her own bank account.

After I left Caroline's room that day, my mind raced. How could I help her, since she could not even hire me? I contacted the attorneys who told me there was nothing they could do. I asked for suggestions. One told me to contact her guardian *ad litem*, an attorney appointed by the court to protect her rights and advocate for her. He told me to report her present conditions to the guardian's attorney, who was the eldest son who lived in Canada.

When I called the attorney and told him that I was a nurse advocate and wanted to report that she was a victim of medical negligence and wanted the guardianship removed since she was clearly mentally competent, he started to scream at me and accuse me of HIPPA violations. He told me in no uncertain terms to stay away from her and to have no further contact with her. I got off the phone after politely asking him to please tell her son that she was in a terrible situation and needed to get into a better place soon. The attorney sounded very unconcerned for the patient's dire straits. I was stunned. What was going on here?

I decided to go to her next court hearing to see what I could learn. Before I went, I sought counsel from one of the best guardianship/mental health attorneys in Chicago. He told me what typically happened at hearings on guardianship matters and advised me to be a very quiet fly on the wall if I were to observe the open court hearing. What I saw in court confirmed my suspicions: her sons likely did not have her financial best interests in mind. Her son's attorney portrayed the family as very devoted and concerned for her welfare, but asked permission to sell one of her properties to pay for her long-term care needs. All three of her sons, who had visited once in the previous six months were portrayed as devoted and concerned for her best interests. Something did not fit.

I went home wondering what was true. Was Caroline really being imprisoned against her will by sons who wanted full access to her finances, hoping that she would die in the low-quality nursing home so that they would inherit the $1,750,000 that she was worth? Why would professional children raised by a single mother not visit her, yell at her on the phone, and threaten never to speak to her again if she did not go along with the guardianship? If Caroline was right, this was one of the saddest cases of family betrayal that I had ever seen.

One positive thing that came out of the court hearing was that Caroline was permitted to request an attorney of her own choosing; she asked for my colleague — one of the top attorneys in Chicago. This was a highly unusual request coming from a person who had been painted by her family as experiencing mental illness.

I could tell that everyone in the room was shocked at her bold request, and they all looked at each other and kindly told Caroline, "In case he cannot accept your case, is it okay if we choose another for you?" She told the judge that this would be okay. Imagine the shock when my friend's partner accepted the case a few minutes later outside the courtroom.

While there are many cases when guardianship must be pursued when patients leave no instructions to family members regarding their wishes, there are always people out there who will take advantage of their parents when they are at their weakest and most vulnerable.

This case kept me up at night, praying and hoping to find ways to help this poor woman. I will admit that I refused to heed the advice of her son's attorney. I continued to visit her, talk to her daily on the phone, and help on the sidelines. Until the day she was released from her captivity and once again able to be captain of her own ship, I would not stop. I am beginning to understand why our state needs a department of elder abuse and adult protective services. Unfortunately, they are some of the most overworked and under-appreciated heroes of our state government.

Not all cases that look like this turn out to be actual cases of elder abuse and neglect, though. I respect and admire attorneys who work in the industry and can weed out truth from fiction. On more than one occasion, I have been wrong about a sad story that turned out to be a mentally unwell patient weaving a tall tale. In this business, truth is often far stranger than fiction. In most cases, the U.S. justice system works, though more slowly than some of us wish.

Several months into this case, I unfortunately learned the whole story. Caroline did, in fact, have a history of two forms of severe mental illness, along with early dementia. She had not told us the truth in entirety. Ultimately, she refused to comply with appropriate treatment and we had to go through the process of extricating ourselves from the case. Sometimes, things are not what they appear to be, but we have learned valuable lessons along the way. Our personal responses when encountering suspected cases of elder abuse must always be cautious and thoughtful with the intention being to help. Advocating for those who cannot advocate for themselves does not always turn out the way we expect, but ethically it seems the best course of action, in most cases.

Tips to Equip: Prepare for the possibility that you may become incapacitated

3. **Take the time and make the investment:** have legal papers drawn up to enforce your wishes. It's not enough to write down your wishes and get it notarized. There must be legally binding documents in place. Only a legal expert in this field will know how to ensure your wishes are respected if you are no longer able to advocate on your own behalf.

4. As you have your legal documents drawn up, **be sure to differentiate the assignment for your healthcare and your finances** (more on this in the *Documents and Insurance* chapter). **Periodically review the documents you have**

drawn up to ensure they reflect your current wishes and not the wishes you had 10 years ago. Those wishes may not reflect the existence of your designee, nor your current relationship.

Chapter 10

Options for Senior Living

In recent years, the number of high-quality skilled nursing facilities (SNFs or nursing homes) has dwindled due to the reduction in reimbursement rates by Medicare. The ones who are most in demand often have long waiting lists. For Medicaid patients, the options are even fewer. It's a tangled web out there, and my focus is usually to keep our senior clients out of hospitals and nursing homes as much as possible. A little prevention and careful attention to small details can make a big difference for seniors. The food at SNFs is not always what individuals want to eat, and their rates of infection can be quite high, so we like to explore all options before making this decision with our clients. With a private healthcare advocate on their team, some patients can remain at home with nursing care, enjoying the comforts of their own home and food. For those who are unable to afford the private pay of having a PPHA and a high-quality home care company that the care manager nurse oversees, we refer them to community organizations that can make referrals.

The cost of care in assisted living and skilled nursing facilities is inexpensive, and Medicare doesn't pay for long-term care in assisted-living or SNFs. The only time Medicare pays for SNF care is after a hospitalization, and it is only for a maximum of 100 days. According to a 2011 survey by Met Life, the national average cost for basic services in an assisted living facility is $41,724 a year, and for a nursing home it's $78,110 for a semi-private room and

$87,235 for a private room.

We have discussed the growing population of the Sandwich Generation in a previous chapter, so we are already aware that many of us will find ourselves, at some point, forced to suggest or encourage our parent(s) to move into a safer place. Investing in your parents' care and support as they age is never a bad idea. The reasons to be concerned for their safety are numerous, but most often attached to memory problems. Most people, when hearing the words "memory loss," immediately think of Alzheimer's disease. While Alzheimer's disease is the most common type of dementia, it is not the only one. The memory loss may also be normal aging (what many call "senior moments," such as forgetting someone's name), MCI (mild cognitive impairment), vascular dementia, a thyroid condition, a head injury, or a medication side effect that is causing the change in cognition. To get a definitive reason for the decline, the patient will need to see a neurologist for testing. It may not be an easy task to get the person with cognitive decline to a neurologist; it is a very delicate issue, and it may take time to convince them to get tests done at all. They may be in denial of how serious the memory issues have become. It's also possible that they are (understandably) totally frightened at the possibility of Alzheimer's disease. You can often couch the issue of the neurologist's visit within the fact that there are many treatable reasons for memory loss. Explain that the only way to find those treatable causes is to go see the physician and be evaluated. Regardless of the reason for the memory loss, the focus still needs to remain around the issue of safety.

Many families are often afraid to broach the subject of mental impairment as they watch their parents age. Confronting a loved one about their memory issues often brings up feelings of betrayal, denial, anger and embarrassment for the person with the memory loss, and guilt for the adult children or spouse. Let's face it: it would be difficult to admit to your loved ones that you have lost your ability to safely live alone. Memory loss often happens slowly and people tend to hide the signs.

Unless you spend a significant amount of time with your parents or grandparents, it can be months or even years before the harsh reality hits. Seniors are often resistant to moving; they feel that going into a senior living community constitutes a surrender of one's independence and dignity, and signifies the end of the road. The reality is that many assisted and independent living communities are far from depressing! They have all the amenities of home, and many conveniences that make life much easier and safer for seniors. Sadly, the decision to delay a move can be a dangerous one. Remember: if you fail to plan, you plan to fail. It is tragic when an accident or other medical calamity makes the decision an urgent and even more stressful one.

If you notice a senior in your life is becoming more and more forgetful, the best thing to do is have a family meeting without your senior loved one before there is a crisis. The purpose of the meeting is to plan a unified and loving approach to the discussion of moving. If there is a unified consensus and a willingness to help all around, the move will be much easier, with no hurt feelings on anyone's part. The message should be a clear and loving one: "Mom, we love you too much to see you live alone any longer. If you fall, or if anything dangerous happens, we would be heartbroken. We see how you are struggling (give examples here), and we all agree that the time has come to choose a better living situation."

After you and the rest of the family present the idea of moving, let the parent or couple speak and ask as many questions as possible. It is important that they know they are respected and are being heard. Oftentimes, they will admit that they need help. Sometimes, they won't be ready to have the conversation and will react with anger. If that should happen, save it for another day and another gentle conversation.

They may be resistant to moving due to the daunting task of moving itself. Moving is overwhelming to most of us, but especially if you are elderly, have a lifetime of things with memories in your home, and are living in a body that doesn't physically feel up to the task of sorting, tossing, and packing. The good news is that if everyone pitches in, it can be manageable. If everyone is not willing or able to pitch in, and there are financial resources available, there are many "senior move specialist" services available that will handle everything — from sorting through belongings to packing, from hiring the mover to arranging the handyman to fix up the residence prior to putting it up for sale, from shuttling away old items to donation centers to setting up belongings at the new home.

Independent Senior Living Facilities

When asked, many seniors will say that they would prefer to stay in their own home, with assistance as needed. Moving to a smaller home, such as an apartment or a condo with the financial resources for a caregiver, may be a great option. Keep in mind that 24-hour caregivers are very expensive; even at a very meager rate of $12 an hour privately, you are still looking at spending over $5000 to $7000 a month for 24-hour care, plus "nanny taxes" that you will have to pay. Home care agencies are often the safest and highest-quality option, but hourly rates are often $26 or more per hour. Don't forget to add in the usual living expenses that we all have. There are other options for independent senior living, and those would be found in senior retirement communities. Independent senior living might be appropriate for someone with very early Alzheimer's disease or dementia who can still live independently, but can't manage an entire house. In these communities, seniors live in apartments of varying square footage with a tiny kitchen (because it isn't used much), and residents go to a restaurant-style community dining room for most of their meals. There are buses for transportation around town, and plenty of time for activities and socialization, which is excellent for someone with mild cognitive decline.

Senior living communities may be on a rental-by-the-month basis, or they may be part of a "continuing care community" where there is a buy-in fee. The advantage of rental communities is that loved ones can move from one community to another without financial penalty. For example, when an adult child gets a job transfer from Michigan to Arizona, her elderly dad can move from his senior rental community near his daughter in Michigan to one close to where his daughter is moving to in Arizona, keeping the two of them close together at all times. Independent senior communities often also offer assisted living if that should become necessary. How would you know if it's time to move for a loved one to move to assisted living? The crucial factors mostly boil down to two: memory and mobility. If you need help getting up, or with taking your medication, it's time for assisted living. Even in senior independent living, staff will still unobtrusively monitor the condition of the resident's apartment; whether they're grooming themselves and/or acting appropriately; how much they're eating; and any atypical behaviors are reported and monitored in weekly staff meetings. So even in independent living communities, there is oversight by staff for the purposes of safety.

Senior continuing care retirement communities, better known as CCRCs

To move into a CCRC, there is a buy-in fee which can vary in price (depending on the place) from roughly $100,000 to over $1 million. In addition to the buy-in fee, you will often also pay a monthly fee to live there. The advantage of a continuing care community is that even if you run out of money, they will continue to care for you and allow you to live there for the rest of your life.

Continuing care communities typically offer a full spectrum of living situations: *independent senior living, assisted living, memory care, and a skilled nursing facility.* One caveat is that the CCRC or "Life Care" community will decide where you belong within their facility. Even if you don't feel ready for the skilled nursing facility, that is where you'll be living if the administration there decides that's where you belong. The savvy shopper at a CCRC will probably wonder: what happens if I die a month after I move in? Am I out the huge buy-in that I paid last month? The answer can vary. Some CCRCs offer a "money back" buy-in fee (typically higher than the "no money back" fee; you then have the option of moving out or getting buy-in money back when you die). Do your homework before signing on the bottom line for a CCRC. Couples hardly ever age at the same rate. Have an attorney look over the contract carefully. They are a big investment, but with potential for a lot of long-term security with the assurance of lifetime care.

Assisted Living Facilities

Assisted living is an intermediate between independent living and a skilled nursing facility. They are typically staffed 24 hours a day, and residents can choose what level of assistance they'd like (such as assistance with dressing, bathing, meals, or medication reminders). The federal government does not regulate assisted-living facilities. Costs for assisted living will vary by the facility, and not all of them are set up specifically for patients with memory loss. You need to ask the right questions when checking out these facilities (Alzheimer's Association, 2016).

Memory Care Facilities

It seems that on nearly every corner, a memory care facility, sometimes referred to as a special care unit, is being built. There is a growing need for these facilities; many people are living longer and with increasing age, there are increasing numbers of persons with Alzheimer's disease. Statistically, 38 percent of persons 85 years of age have Alzheimer's disease and 1 in 9 elderly persons has Alzheimer's disease. Many nursing homes also offer memory care in a special care unit where patients with memory loss are grouped together. Staff in special care units should be specifically trained in memory care, offer activities for persons with memory challenges, and be skilled in handling behavioral issues (Alzheimer's Association, 2016). Many states require special care units to disclose what type of specialized care they offer; please ask for their Special Care Unit Disclosure form when you visit for more information.

Skilled Nursing Facilities

If your or your loved one does require skilled nursing care

that is beyond the scope of assisted living, it can be daunting to think about where to start looking. Did you know that Medicare doesn't pay for long-term care in a skilled nursing facility? They will only pay for 100 days, per year, of short-term rehabilitation after a hospitalization; afterwards, the cost falls on the patient. If you don't have money for the SNF, you will need to apply for Medicaid—and then find a good nursing home that accepts Medicaid. Some good news is that the medicare.gov website has some helpful resources to help you select a skilled nursing facility (better known as a SNF, pronounced "sniff" by healthcare professionals). First, at the Medicare website, check out the SNF checklist (www.medicare.gov/files/skilled-nursing-facility-checklist.pdf).

The SNF Checklist is a document composed of a series of yes-or-no questions to be answered as you visit each skilled nursing facility (SNF). You will need to print a separate checklist for each SNF you're planning to visit. The questions are designed to evaluate the quality of the nursing home, and to help you decide if this facility might be a good fit for you personally. Many of the questions on the checklist are ones you may not think to ask on your own. If you visit a facility that seems to fit your needs, it's a good idea to place your name on the waiting list even if you're not sure you want to move your loved one there. Many of the good facilities have long waiting lists. Ask what happens if your loved one runs out of money; do they accept Medicaid? You'll also want to check out "Nursing Home Compare" at the Medicare website (www.medicare.gov/nhcompare/). Use the nursing home comparison information, and combine that with the information gathered on your visits and recorded on your SNF Checklist to help you find a SNF that is of good quality and a good fit for your loved one.

It is common for families to struggle with the decision of whether it is the right thing to do to place their loved one in a residential facility. We've adapted these questions from the Alzheimer's Association to get you thinking. (Alzheimer's Association, 2016)_

Tips to Equip: When to consider alternate living arrangements

1. Is my loved one becoming unsafe in their current home?
2. Is the health of the person or my health as a caregiver at risk?
3. Are the person's care needs beyond my physical abilities?
4. Am I becoming a stressed, irritable and impatient caregiver?
5. Am I neglecting work responsibilities, my family and myself?
6. Would the structure and social interaction at a care facility benefit the person with the health issues?

It is normal to feel a wide range of emotions when placing your loved one in any type of facility after living in their own home. Most families find it best to make the decision and swiftly move forward. The safety of our loved one is at stake, and the risks are just too great not to act. This is something we enjoy helping families navigate more easily, as it is frightening and frustrating for everyone. Often, aging parents may listen to professionals in ways they will not listen to their own families. It's all in how the message is presented, and it must be presented with compassion and fairness to all in a loving, respectful manner.

Chapter 11

Exploring Alternative Therapies

This chapter explores alternative therapies as a method of treating many ailments. While Western medicine remains prevalent in modern healthcare, there are too many cases where holistic doctors have helped patients manage pain and recover from illness to discount this method of healthcare. Integrative medicine physicians often focus more on prevention of medical calamities through diet, proper exercise, chiropractic care, and Eastern medicine modalities.

Many major medical centers around the country are now combining conventional Western medicine with alternative or complementary treatments such as naturopathic supplements; acupuncture; massage; biofeedback; yoga; meditation; stress reduction; and organic nutritional support. The holistic model of care aims to treat the whole person instead of just the disease. Traditional Western medicine proponents refer to this approach as "complementary" to emphasize that such treatments are used *with* mainstream medicine, not as replacements or alternatives.

The American Hospital Association notes that the number of hospitals that offer complementary therapies has more than tripled in the last decade, and more hospitals are planning to add complementary therapies and/or departments (AHA.org). Several studies show that these therapies can greatly reduce unpleasant symptoms associated with chemotherapy. They reduce pain, nausea, anxiety, and even promote healing in post-surgical patients.

Cancer Treatment Centers of America is one well-known proponent of integrative medicine. Their surgeons and oncologists routinely work side-by-side with staff naturopaths and pharmacists to make certain that patients receive a full array of complementary modalities. Acupuncture, massage, chiropractic care, Reiki therapy and even laughter therapy are offered at CTCA by the mind-body medicine department. A large pastoral care team makes certain that all patients have support to pray and meditate as they heal, and superior patient satisfaction is cited year after year (cancercenter.com).

Northwestern Memorial Hospital is another well-known major medical center that is known for its cutting-edge integrative medicine department, as well as Duke University and hundreds of other centers around the country that recognize the huge impact that integrative medicine has in our society. The Oster Center for Integrative Medicine in San Francisco at the University of California has joined with Harvard, Columbia, and dozens of other academic medical centers to form the Consortium of Academic Health Centers for Integrative Medicine.

Danny McLane is a Doctor of Chiropractic Medicine and practices in Northern Illinois. Many people do not realize how much more chiropractors do than make spinal adjustments to help manage pain. I think their real value is in their vast knowledge of integrative health. By integrative, I mean nontraditional methods to heal the human body: things like chiropractic adjustments, acupuncture, Reiki, massage therapy, ultrasonic treatments, and most importantly, nutrition. Nutrition is a gift to the human body. People who eat well and exercise have tapped into the best possible way to support the body's innate ability to heal itself. Traditional methods may fail to bring actual healing, and many people come to Danny "when all else fails."

Why not start the healing process with the safest, lowest-risk, and most effective way to bring about natural healing first? I have seen firsthand what non-traditional methods can do. Osteopathic physicians and doctors of chiropractic medicine have much more training in nutrition and spinal pathology than medical doctors. They help people avoid dangerous cocktails of high-risk medicines that may do more harm than good when they are used carelessly.

Alternative Medicine – A Different Perspective

By Danny McLane

Integrative medicine, holistic medicine, natural medicine… so many ways to describe taking care of the body in a way that is complementary to how the body heals itself, in most cases, without any need for Western medicine.

When Teri asked me to write my perspective on Integrative Medicine, I thought, "Sure, but it will be like a drop of water in the ocean." Since we have just a chapter to get into a very broad and deep topic, let's jump on in.

I do not oppose the current standard of Western medical care, even though I may sound contrary to that in the next few statements. What I am contrary to is dogma: accepting the current model just because it's been accepted or because we've become accustomed to it. The use of over-the-counter (OTC) medications is incredibly prevalent. One recent report by Information Resources Inc. (IRI) stated that in 2015 there were 2.9 billion trips to retail outlets to buy OTC meds. These medications offer people the ability to reduce their pain and their symptoms. Some of these medications even allow people to *recover* from the minor issues that caused them to turn to OTCs in the first place. In many houses all over the country, if you look for a medicine cabinet, you're sure to find one; it's a common standard.

Then there's prescription medication, which has to be prescribed by a doctor. Those are fairly common as well, especially in the instance of the need for drugs that address common conditions. These drugs can range from statins for cholesterol to something more extreme, such as chemotherapy drugs for cancer. We often see the concept of "a pill for any ill" in practice, but has this concept gotten out of hand? I don't think so. I know many well-intentioned doctors who have their heart and head in the right place, which is squarely in line with the best interest of their patients. It's my opinion that we're missing a step in the process. First, let's assess the risks versus the benefits to the patient, because *all* medications have side effects.

How bad can it be?

Pretty bad, it turns out. According to the Centers for Disease Control, poisoning by drugs is the number one cause of injury-related death in the United States. That includes taking (or giving) too much of a substance that was not intended to cause harm.

Let that sink in.

The reality is, drugs kill more people every year than you can imagine. An estimated 280,000 people die from accidental drug-related deaths every year, and these are not illegal narcotics we're talking about. This is not meant to shock you, but to help shift your perspective. Paracelsus, the father of toxicology, is most memorably noted for saying, "The dose makes the poison."

In our modern culture we simply take too many drugs. Let me rephrase that: we rely on drugs to solve problems that they should not be relied upon for. How do we know? Even though America is less than the five percent of the world's total population, we consume 80 percent of opioid painkillers produced in the world. Couple that fact with the fact that, despite having the most expensive healthcare in the world, medical error is the third leading cause of death in America for at least the last 12 years running. Our quality of healthcare ranks at #25, according to the World Health Organization.

Let's talk about some commonly-prescribed OTC medications. There is a whole classification of drugs that are called non-steroidal anti-inflammatories (NSAIDS). They make up most of what people buy and use for common aches and pains of everyday life. Things like lower back pain, headaches, neck pain and so on. Something so mundane should be easily handled by what we've been using, right? The answer is a double-edged sword.

In a study done with over 114,000 teachers in California, the evidence shows that there was an increased risk of breast cancer from daily use of ibuprofen or aspirin over five years. For ibuprofen the risk increased by 50 percent… and for aspirin, the risk increased by 80 percent. The pills reduce pain, but increase the risk of breast cancer.

This classification of drugs carries with it a significant risk of heart-related death as well. What's worse: the increased risks were not related to lengthy periods of time for the use of the drug, either. There have been studies that reported that people taking the drugs for at least six months were dying at twice the rate of others who were not taking them. The risk was the worst with people who used ibuprofen. They die at three times the rate of non-NSAID users. That's a 200 to 300 percent increased risk of death from heart attack, stroke, or other heart-related problem.

I realize that this is all a little shocking, but in reality, it's only a symptom of a sick system. In fairness, they are doing the best they can with what they have. They, the people, are saving lives. But why, then, are people so sick, so lost, so disappointed?

Most disease is a natural reaction to an unnatural environment.

I know I hit the facts pretty hard up front, but bear with me. I have a few stories to share to illustrate my point, and I think that you'll enjoy them.

Jessie was a woman in her early forties. She had a robust fervor for life. She took college classes, not because she wanted to get a degree, but to challenge her mind. She worked out six days a week to keep her body fit and healthy. She was a health food enthusiast, who kept her house and her diet clean. She had a loving husband and daughter. She was the model of health... until she wasn't healthy anymore. Her cancer set in suddenly and without warning. Jessie's health degraded very quickly. She sought out the very best in medical care, drew her family close and did everything she could to survive.

Ben, on the other hand, was a man in his late fifties. He was a little overweight, but not unhealthy. He had a busy life as a computer programmer. He never paid much attention to what he ate or to exercise. One aspect that he did get right was time off. He often took vacations with his wife and children. His health predicament started when his right hand stopped working. In fact, everything from his shoulder to his first row of knuckles on his right hand stopped functioning altogether. Nothing seemingly caused it. When Ben came to my office, he'd already been "everywhere." He told me that he tried everything. "Everything" cost him eight months and $10,000. He still didn't know what caused it, or how to fix it. His wife made sure that he had the best medical attention to help him solve his problem. Everything from nerve testing, CT scans and MRIs. The doctors found nothing. By all accounts he should have been able to move his arm freely, yet he couldn't. He was losing hope. He wasn't nearly as hopeless as another man I treated.

When Jeff came into my office, he wasn't looking for a treatment for himself. He had already resigned himself to a life of pain. He was there accompanying his daughter, who hurt her back practicing golf. She had aspirations of becoming a professional golfer. Her parents wanted the absolute best for her, and were coming to see me as a last resort. They didn't like the options that her orthopedist gave her. The physical therapy they had already tried didn't help. During the interview, we started down a line of conversation that eventually led to us talking about Jeff and his back. He was training his daughter because he had been very good at golf, before his back went out. As you can imagine, Jeff had lost hope for his condition. He was there for his daughter; he never really asked if I could help him. He just assumed that it was too late for him to have a normal life. He was plagued by extreme fatigue. He had enough energy to get up brush his teeth, get dressed and go downstairs; but before he could prepare breakfast for himself, he had to stop between the bedroom and the kitchen for a nap to get his energy back. Imagine the mental pain and loss of hope this man had, which brings to my next topic that we need to cover, for frame of reference.

The psychology of illness.

One of the greatest quotes on optimism came from a politician who had just recently taken office as the mayor of Orange County, California. She said, "Just because we've destroyed 90 percent of everything, doesn't mean we can't do amazing things with the remaining 10 percent." What she was talking about was maintaining optimism in the face of a broken-down system. There was an obvious spin to her comment. She was trying to emphasize the little positive that was left.

Buckminster Fuller, the father of modern nanotechnology, has been quoted as saying, "You never change things by fighting the existing reality. To change something, build a new model that makes the existing model obsolete."

The psychology of illness prevents us from finding a proper solution. It also encourages us to accept the standard of living that we see all around us. The number of times that I hear somebody attributing a breakdown in his or her body to normal aging is staggering. Many studies on conformity in a social setting show us just this. People tend to think that what is common is normal. It tells me that, as a population, we have a perception problem.

What if we stop simply accepting whatever our traditional doctor tells us is the only solution?

What if we do nothing? This is a normal option that I offer to my patients all the time. In fact, doing nothing is the right option for treating certain conditions. My professor of radiology used to call certain x-ray findings "leave me alone" lesions. Referring to the best method of care was to ignore it. But is that the best option in this case? I say no.

My massage therapy instructor always used to harp on us. Every class. He'd say, "If the only tool you have is a hammer, every problem looks like a nail, and you won't know what to do with a screw! Get more tools in your tool box." Seriously, every class we heard this. It made me constantly ask questions, some of which I didn't even need an answer for at the time. It served me later on in my career and in my personal life. I found the courage to ask questions as well as seek more options. It os often safest to start with the least dangerous, most natural options first. If those don't work, keep looking and be open to non-traditional approaches.

The first question most people want to ask is, "What are my alternatives?" I know it took a while to get to the good stuff. Everyone wants to jump right in to what integrative medicine has to offer, without knowing why it's so important. Please forgive me if you had already come to that conclusion without my preamble. In Chinese medicine, they ask the question, "Can you eat bitter? Can you endure the bitter, so you'll recognize the sweetness?" If you were to ask about the alternatives first, you would have missed another step.

So many disciplines of medicine skip ahead to the fancy, exotic stuff and overlook the basics. To miss the small stuff is to miss the big stuff. This is *my* perspective, because as a chiropractic doctor, we spend the majority of our time learning how the body is supposed to work. We master the basics. We do this so that we can notice when it's not functioning properly. Once we find it, we can define it and start our work to solve these issues. This approach is vitally important to medicine. A problem well-defined; is a problem half-solved. What you can do is look to the common things of everyday life first, and make sure that they are in order.

The Big Idea.

The body is a self-healing, self-regulating organism. It makes no mistakes, but has limitations, which is the most important frame of reference you can have when approaching health. B.J. Palmer, who developed chiropractic medicine, called it the 'Big Idea.' He was known to say, "Get the big idea, and everything else will follow."

Our body will do what it does, so long as there is no interference. This interference comes in the form of negative thoughts, traumas, toxins, extreme temperature, and self-inflicted abuse. We all know thoughts and feelings can help heal, or hurt. Physical traumas can leave a lifelong burden on our body unless properly cared for. These injuries can be acute, such as a fall or crash; or chronic, as in poor posture or repeated misuse of a joint. Injuries can also be a side effect of a life-saving procedure. Surgical scars impact the tissue for years afterwards. Toxins can be obvious, like lead or cigarette smoke; or insidious, as with recycled water or plastics; temperature is usually pretty obvious. Without the destructive force of interference, the body usually heals naturally.

The innate intelligence of the body knows exactly how to grow a kidney, or repair a damaged eyeball, or digest your food, yet sometimes this doesn't happen. The question is why. If you want to build a brick house, you need bricks. You also need a bricklayer. Otherwise you either have a pile of bricks or a guy standing around without supplies. In order to build a healthy body, it requires good nutrition/chemical building blocks (structure) and properly working physiology (function).

If the limitation on health and growth is chemical (structural) in nature, as in poor nutrition, health will suffer. This is beautifully showcased in the documentary *Fat, Sick and Nearly Dead* (2011). The subject of the documentary, Joe, was very successful in life, but he had poor health. His body was struggling for health because he lacked the raw materials for basic cell function and repair. He recovered his health by drinking juiced vegetables and fruit. As he nourished his body, the limitations on his health resolved and he healed.

If the limitation on health and growth is physiologic (functional) in nature, as seen when a person has a bone out of place that presses on a spinal nerve, causing it to dysfunction, health will also suffer. Standard medical science shows that nerve interference can affect every function in the body. Proper nerve function is how the brain keeps the body functioning. It's almost scary to realize that pressure equal to the weight of a dime, 2.28g, can cause a nerve to dysfunction by 60 percent.

The intent of this work is not to be an exhaustive walk through all of Integrative Medicine, but a glimpse as to what else is available to you and your loved ones seeking health. Now that we have the Big Idea, let's build on it.

When we look at the body as healing and self-regulating, food comes to mind as an obvious starting point, right? Actually, the most important starting point is the control center of the body, which is the nervous system. It controls and coordinates every function in the body. Simply stated, everyone needs to get checked and corrected by a chiropractor because we are specialized in restoring proper function to the nervous system.

The job of the nervous system is to adapt our bodies to the stresses we encounter in everyday life. Without it, we die. Without the nervous system functioning at optimal levels, we simply can't function at our best. That means every system within the body suffers: the heart, lungs, immune and digestive systems, muscles, bones, joints, nerves, every single cell. To ensure you are working with all the odds in your favor, I recommend enlisting the help of a chiropractor.

The simplest, most accurate comment about food that I have heard is the following: "Eat food, mostly plants, not too much."

This means you need food. Real food, not food-products. The Standard American Diet (SAD) is comprised of 63 percent empty calories with no nutritional benefit. It is no wonder people are sick with any manner of lifestyle disease.

There is no such thing as health food or junk food. There is food, and then there is junk. Just because you *can* eat it, doesn't mean you *should*. All real food is health food. If it's not food, it's junk. The body is resilient, so people can get away with eating junk for a long time. The body will compensate as much as it can, for as long as it can. Once it can't, it won't. Unfortunately, by the time symptoms of poor health show up, all the back up plans have been exhausted, and the body has entered into a state of "biological debt." The answer lies in eating well. This is the second most important thing you can do for your health.

What about eating well *and* drinking well? Do you drink enough water?

Water is the universal solvent. It dissolves and carries the majority of chemistry we need to perform most biological functions in the body. You need water for that. The only way the food we eat gets to where it's going in our body is by a river of blood. You need water for that. When we eat a full meal, our body uses the fluid from our blood, about 75 percent of the total volume, for digestion. Most of that water is added in the form of saliva and digestive juices. Then it's reabsorbed in the colon. You need water for that. A general guideline for a healthy individual is 2 to 2.5 liters of water per day, plus enough to offset any diuretics, such as coffee, tea and alcohol. Dehydration can be defined as a one percent or greater loss of body mass due to fluid loss.

Movement is an important key to life. Blood flows out to the body from the heart in order to sustain life. This is an active pump. The return of blood from the body to the heart is passive. The same is true for the lymphatic fluid. Your lymphatic system acts as a sewer in the body, draining off the waste. This is also true of the fluid that nourishes our joints—all of them. The same goes for our fluid that nourishes the brain and spinal system. All of these systems are only effective at cleaning and feeding the body when it moves. The bowels have some natural motion, but are aided greatly when the body, as a whole, moves. The heart is one muscular pump. All the other muscles play the role of muscular pump for all the other fluids.

So it makes perfect sense to assume that anything that keeps you moving is good for your health. We see that evidenced by scientific studies; they show that exercise is beneficial for sleep, memory, strength, power, balance, functionality, reduced pain, lower blood pressure, reduced psychiatric symptoms, and really? This list could keep going. These are but a small fraction of how exercise helps the body and mind stay healthy. If ever there was a doubt, it should be clear by now that exercise is a key to health. In the book *Younger Next Year*, Chris Crowley and Henry S. Lodge, M.D., discuss how living with health as a mindset can reverse the biological effects of aging. This is true. In my clinic, I see youthful elderly and aged youth. I also regularly witness the recovery of function that was lost to "normal aging." As we covered before, interference affects us all and diminishes our total capacity. So be aware that many signs or complaints that gather as one ages, are simply due to lack of proper maintenance. The body will heal if it is given what it needs.

Time is a catalyst; it allows you to do more of what you are doing. If the impact of your choices is negative, your health becomes more negative. When you start choosing more healthful options, your health recovers. This is where many people get stuck. It happens to everyone: "but I've been doing it for years" and "it's never made a difference before" are phrases commonly used when someone denies a bad habit that is taking away their health.

Imagine that you are in an airplane, cruising at 30,000 feet. If you lose 1000 feet, not much of anything happens. However, if you repeat that drop in altitude every 10 minutes, the effects will be more tangible. If the windows on the plane were covered, you wouldn't realize there was an issue until the landing gear of the plane started hitting the tops of the tallest trees. In health, this is when symptoms start. Not at the beginning, when you first lose altitude, but near the end, just before a crash. Be proactive. Start now. Get time on your side.

In healthcare, there are options. Many times, there is a rift between what you will be told in a hospital setting and the Complementary and Alternative Medicine (CAM) setting. This rift is simply a lack of understanding. The science is all there. I will lay out for you a few examples, out of literally thousands, where the CAM treatments are the best option. Not just in terms of safety, but *real* results. Sometimes you can be your own guru and find these options for yourself. But many times, you need an expert to navigate the complexities of options availed to you.

Teri and I agree that the best way to help people is to empower and equip them. It's one of the many reasons I respect her approach. She does a wonderful job helping people understand not only what can be done, but what *else* can be done. This is one of the reasons I offer a free daily health update to all my clients. A well-informed patient is one who can help themselves. It puts power in the hands of people who want to be healthy.

There is danger in stopping the search for the best healthcare solution. There is a phenomenon that happens in regular people, not just doctors, nurses, and healthcare workers, called search satisfaction. It is the tendency of a person to stop searching once they find a solution. This is a great help if you're looking for a lost set of keys, but it can be outright disastrous in healthcare. Why? Any help will help, but the right help, in the right way, will help the most. A human is not a standardized unit.

There exists a significant amount of variability in people and the way they function. So how does this apply? In, *The 7 Habits of Highly Effective People,* the author, Stephen Covey, uses the phrase "nothing fails like success." His implication is that success doesn't generalize out of context. What works for one person may not work for another. Oftentimes, it will not work for the *same* person at a different time.

To correlate that perspective to search satisfaction, the picture that starts to form is a grim one. We go back to the saying, "If the only tool you have is a hammer, every problem looks like a nail." This is one of the biggest problems in healthcare that integrative medicine addresses. When people get hurt, they want a solution. They trust their doctors to lead them to the best option. And doctors do, don't they? In a huge study of workers with back pain, that answer became very clear. Of people who went to a surgeon, 42.7 percent had back surgery. Of people who went to a Doctor of Chiropractic, 1.5 percent had surgery.

This isn't to imply that surgeons are bad doctors. Not at all. They are great doctors. They are great at what they do, but they are not always great at what they don't do. There's an old adage in healthcare: "What you're not up on, you're down on." Basically, you endorse and support what you know.

That's great if you are looking to buy a new pair of shoes, or for recommendations for a good restaurant in town. But this is major. Every doctor takes an oath that begins: "First, do no harm." No one is going to argue that a life-saving surgery comes with acceptable risks, but what about a less invasive, safer way to solve the same problem? Remember, drugs are not without danger either. In 2010, 38,329 people died from pharmaceutical drugs or prescription opioid drugs. Compare that to chiropractic care: during the course of about 100 clinical trials, not a single patient experienced a major adverse side effect. This is only to emphasize that other options are available and should be used first. You can always get multiple opinions before making your choice.

Confidence in an inadequate solution prevents participation in an adequate solution.

Options limit choices and choices limit outcomes. Now that we have come this far into our time together, let's look back and see the finality of the three stories we started earlier on in the chapter. We have a clearer perspective as to why integrative healthcare is essential.

Jeff, the gentleman who had back pain but was more concerned about his daughter… let's start with him. He had lost hope for his back pain because he was told he couldn't be helped. He had a panel of nine specialists at a prestigious hospital system review his case. These specialists did everything they knew to do, to help him. They sent him to a bigger, even more prestigious hospital for further testing and evaluation. They told him the same message. They gave him a diagnosis of Transverse Myelitis. TM is usually only found at one nerve level, and only on one side of the body. Jeff had it at every level, on both sides. I agreed with the "-itis» part of his diagnosis. He was certainly inflamed. So I dug in deeper. I did something radical and I asked him what he ate. None of his other doctors talked to Jeff about food. He told me that because of his condition he ate whatever his wife made for dinner and some easy things throughout the day. He used the term junk food. I corrected him. "Jeff, it's just junk, there's no food in that," I said. He agreed to make a significant change in his diet, mostly because he was desperate and it was a change that both he and his daughter needed, but I kept digging.

I asked him what hobbies he was involved in, what sports he played, and if he had a history of injury. It was messy. He had an extensive history with a lot of suspect behaviors. All that could have caused his issues. I asked him what he did for a living before he was disabled. He shared that he had been working in an office a few years. He'd had to get an office job after his lower back started to bother him while he was finishing a concrete flooring project. I had a moment when it hit me. I asked what kind of finishing he was doing.

His reply? "Epoxy, mostly."

I had a flashback to my Organic Chemistry 2 class. Epoxides are an extremely volatile and reactive species of compound. They are used in industry to make a reaction happen: a combination of liquids reacts into a solid. He'd been breathing these compounds into his lungs. The nerves that go to the lungs are between the ribs, on both sides, at every level of the thoracic spine. That was it. He had epoxide poisoning. That explained why the adjusting helped, and the massage helped and the pool therapy helped. But none of them solved his issue. He needed a nutritional intervention. Not drugs, not body work. I recommended he watch the documentary *Fat, Sick and Nearly Dead,* and start on vegetable juice right away. He did. In less than three months, he was out golfing again. So he stopped juicing. His pain came back, although, this time not as harsh, so he began again. The pain stopped again. He asked me, "Doc, how long do I have to juice?" I replied, "Does it matter? You're living your life now, right?"

What about Ben? The programmer whose right arm shut off? Who really knows what happened? I set aside about an hour to work with him the first visit because I had no idea how it would go. After he ran down his list of interventions that he tried, and my list of issues which happen commonly, all was but exhausted. So I decided to use Applied Kinesiology (AK) to map out what was functioning and what was not. Now, AK looks odd, because it's not a very well-known technique. Rather than attempting to explain all the intricacies, I just went about my work. It's a system that uses reflex points to help focus the brain on nerve pathways so they function better. Sure enough, after 45 minutes of Ben telling me I was rubbing the wrong spot, that his leg had nothing to do with his shoulder, he proclaimed his need to visit my restroom. When he stood up, he pushed himself up with both hands, and walked to the restroom. Didn't even notice. When he came out, he reached back and swung the door closed, with his right hand. Then looked at me and asked, "Ok, what's next?" Didn't even notice. So I asked, "Hey Ben, what hand did you zip up with?" This request made him focus on his right arm. He raised his hand up, in front of his face and wiggled his fingers around. His face paled; I thought he was going to pass out. He looked at me and asked, "What did you do?" This was in my first few years of practice when I was a bit more spry. I replied, "You asked me to fix your arm, I fixed your arm... TADA! IT'S MAGIC!"

Ben is Catholic. Magic of this kind was voodoo and not acceptable. After that, I tried to explain to him that it was actually advanced neuroscience. But between the disbelief that a guy, with no technology, could solve a problem that the best hospital care didn't, coupled with my foot-in-mouth comment about magic, he wasn't really receptive to any kind of scientific explanation. Not even if it was about how stimulatory and inhibitory neural networks regulated afferent fibers that... nope. I lost him. He went home to his wife, who had extensive training in rehab as an Occupational Therapist, and told her I was a witch doctor.

But what of Jessi? She died. The second round of chemo was too much for her to handle. The first round helped her fight off cancer but left her immune system devastated. It also radicalized her cancer. The chemo killed off all the daughter cells, but made the mother cells more effective at resisting any kind of therapy.

She was my aunt. I love her and I still miss her.

When most of my clients ask me for an alternative to pain meds, they expect that I will give them a recommendation for a watered-down natural option. They expect that my efforts will only result in a shadow of what the heavy-duty pharmaceuticals can deliver. In fact, one of my go-to options is curcumin. It's an herbal extract from turmeric. There are 9,258 scientific studies in the Pubmed. gov database (at the time of this writing) to show its efficacy. It is better at lowering high cholesterol than Atorvastatin; better than corticosteroids for decreasing inflammation; better than Prozac and Imipramine for depressive behavior; better as a blood thinner than Aspirin; better as an anti-inflammatory than aspirin, ibuprofen, sulindac, phenylbutazone, naproxen, indomethacin, diclofenac, dexamethasone, celecoxib, and tamoxifen; 500-100,000 times better than Metformin at treating type 2 diabetes; better than Oxaliplatin as an anti-proliferative cancer drug. The best-known compound for chemotherapy-resistant and radiation-resistant cancers — and that's the short list. That's also just one example of hundreds. Better options are out there.

New knowledge about pathophysiology emerges constantly. The sphere of information changes every six months. It is not a static topic like math. It is constantly changing in major ways. It changes so rapidly that, over time, it's easy to be stuck with yesterday's news, holding in high esteem many conventional wisdoms that have been proven dead wrong. Did you hear about how the FDA reversed its recommendation for a daily aspirin? They cited that the actual harm outweighed the potential benefits. I read between 10-25 articles per day to stay current. I also offer a daily health update to all of my clients for free, so they can stay current as well. In preparing to write this chapter, I pulled from my collection of research articles — about 600 of the most interesting, relevant new bits of news from the world of science and healthcare. Obviously, I can't share even a fraction of them in this small space. So you see, my friends, I have not presented to you a drop of water in the ocean, but instead, the ocean in a drop of water. Explore. Read. Ask questions. Learn and do better next time.

-Danny

Tips to Equip: Considering alternative medicine

1. More respected medical facilities have complementary medicine specialties to work with Western medicine than ever before; **don't be afraid to have the "alternative medicine" discussion with your physician.** Be prepared for resistance from hardcore traditionalists.

2. Never underestimate the importance of good nutrition.

3. Don't be a slave to dogma.

4. Most disease is a natural reaction to an unnatural environment.

5. Some illnesses can be improved by beginning with a change in your perception.

6. Your body has the innate ability to self-regulate and self-heal without interference, but it does have limitations.

7. Water is a universal solvent; sometimes that's all the body needs.

8. Movement is an important key to life.

Chapter 12

The Importance of Having a Plan

Throughout the previous chapters, I've touched on the importance of putting legal documents in place as well as shared some examples of the ill-effects of not keeping your documents up to date. I will delve a little deeper into this subject in the *Legal Documents* section. As hard as it is to tackle, this subject must be addressed. More and more people are suffering medical catastrophes, to the point where they become incompetent and cannot continue making decisions for their own life and welfare. Whether that is due to mental incapacity, medical malaise or even death, the importance of having legal documents in place to carry out your wishes has never been more important. I will discuss how simple and stress-free it can be with the right team in place.

This chapter also gives more insight into the Affordable Care Act of 2010, or Obamacare. As you read further, you will learn more intricacies of legal documents and the different options in modern healthcare as it relates to insurance coverage. There is much to think about, and planning for success has never been more important. With the recent passing of President Trump's tax overhaul, changes to the ACA are expected, though specifics are still emerging. To understand any upcoming changes to health policy, it's still vital to understand current practices and procedures.

One of the most heartbreaking things that happens in hospitals every day is all too common among our elderly patients. You've probably heard about it yourself: an otherwise healthy, active older patient gets admitted to the hospital for a relatively minor ailment and a cascade of events spills over and progresses rapidly. My friend's elderly aunt, at age 94, moved across state lines to be closer to her sister. All went well until she tripped at home and broke her hip. She went to the hospital and couldn't sleep well, so the doctor ordered a sedative that would help her sleep, but it also made her disoriented and confused. When she woke up in the middle of the night, she fell and hit her head and suffered a bleed on her brain due to the blood thinners she was taking. She was ordered to stay on bed rest and soon developed pneumonia and cardiac problems. Soon the treatment for her cardiac problems led to kidney failure. She got so sick she stopped eating.

Once she stopped eating, more things deteriorated and she was transferred to a skilled nursing facility (SNF). The nurse admitting her could see right away that she was fragile and would probably not survive. A Do Not Resuscitate (DNR) order was entered after consulting with the family and she died shortly thereafter.

The point? Seniors do not generally do well in hospitals, as illustrated in earlier stories. Their immune systems are often weaker, they react more easily to medications, and they do not eat well. If you have a loved one in the hospital, make sure a family member is with them to encourage them to eat and drink, offer them snacks, and take them for frequent short walks in the hallways to keep up their strength. Hospitals do not have the staff to give the same level of attention as in days past, and by the time malnutrition or muscle weakness is noticed, the first thing the discharge planner will want to do is send them to rehab or a SNF. The bottom line is that seniors, adults with disabilities, and the mentally ill are often having a harder time than most in navigating modern healthcare. Because providers are receiving lower reimbursement rates for Medicare/Medicaid patients, it is becoming harder for patients to find excellent doctors who are also accepting Medicare patients (never mind Medicaid patients, which many physicians consider to be charity work).

Hospitals and insurance companies, who are receiving lower reimbursement rates, are working hard to recoup their losses to they remain profitable. Since quality of care is not tied closely to future Medicare reimbursement, there are several changes in the industry that hit seniors hard. Perhaps the most common is the 30-day readmissions controversy that is part of the Affordable Care Act. During President Trump's first year in office, he did uphold the 30-day readmission portion of the ACA, so it seems wise to continue to understand what is at play here.

Not a week goes by that I don't hear stories from seniors, those who care for seniors, and even healthcare providers who are fed up with the scam of the inpatient vs. observation status controversy. This major rule, which is part of the Affordable Care Act, is costing seniors billions of dollars annually as they get stuck with bills for stays in rehab facilities that are not covered. They were never actually an inpatient in the hospital that treated them and decided they were too weak to go directly home. The patient is flabbergasted because they thought they were admitted — they slept in the same bed that they would have if they were fully admitted, but they were actually "admitted" under observation status. This cancels their qualification for rehab benefits by Medicare. Emergency room doctors are under heavy pressure to admit every senior they can as an observation patient.

This is a nice way of saying, "We are concerned about you and think you need close watching, so we are going to keep an eye on you to make sure you are well enough to go home." In reality, the patient's bill is higher because many items are not covered under Medicare Part B, which pays for observation or outpatient-type stays. And if the patient goes home after an inpatient admission and returns within 30 days, the hospital is in no hot water from Medicare because they were never technically admitted in the first place. Rehab will only be paid for by Medicare if the patient was a full admission for at least three midnights.

Over and over again we see frail women in their 80s who fall and have a pelvic fracture. If I were an ER physician, I could guess that elderly woman need rehab post-hospital stay, so I would choose to look carefully for diagnoses and codes that would justify a full admission. These women probably spent years paying social security; they earned those benefits, right? I'd think of doing the right thing for the patient. A full admission should be justified if they have an actual diagnosis.

But it's not so easy. Hospitals, many of them very good hospitals, are getting huge fines every year if they have too many 30-day readmissions. Medicare sees that as faulty discharge planning, so they will penalize these hospitals with high rates of readmission—with hundreds of thousands of dollars in fines that will ultimately only drive up the cost of healthcare for everyone. Somebody has to pay for those huge fines, right?

This policy was added in part to cut down on Medicare fraud and deals with the revolving-door syndrome of seniors who were frequently readmitted within the first month after an inpatient admission. Medicare feels that these readmissions are red flags, sending seniors back home too quickly. Too many of these red flags will affect the hospital's quality rating, and the hospital will receive lower reimbursement rates the following year. This can add up to millions of dollars in fines annually.

The scheme that hospitals came up with to reduce their readmission stats involved admitting all questionable senior admissions under observation status. "Observation" hospitalizations are covered under Medicare Part B, which is technically not a "real" hospitalization, so the hospital is not liable to have so many red flags for repetitive inpatient readmissions. The patient usually does not even realize they are admitted under observation status. They go to a regular room and receive the same services as any full-admission patient would. There is a time limit (three midnights) for observation stays before the doctor is called upon to re-evaluate their admission status or discharge them. Currently, over 40 percent of ER patients are admitted under observation status (Medicare.gov). Nurses and physicians are required to document patient status updates more frequently, and the cost of an observation admission is often higher than a regular admission. Medications administered during an observation stay are also not included in the hospital bill, so seniors pay extra for them.

The real problem occurs when a senior becomes so weak during the hospital stay that inpatient rehabilitation is ordered. Medicare will not cover rehab expenses if the patient goes to rehab from an observation stay, as it is technically an outpatient stay and one cannot move from outpatient to acute inpatient rehab and have it paid for by Medicare. This has caused a huge uproar over the past three years, and consumer advocacy groups have lobbied hard to protect seniors from the financial consequences of this ruling. Care managers in hospitals are supposed to keep patients informed about their admission/observation status, and most of them do, but sometimes that critical piece of information gets lost in the shuffle with copies of admission paperwork and discharge forms. Patients should always verify their admission status before transferring to a rehab facility if they do not want to be surprised by a bill from the rehab facility weeks later.

I once had a client whose mother fell into this trap. Her healthy 87-year-old mother fell at home when she tripped over her little dog. At the hospital, and with X-rays confirming that she had broken her hip, the patient had such severe post-operative pain that she did not move unless she had to. She became weaker, lost her appetite, lost weight, and slept constantly after getting frequent pain pills. One week after her surgery, she tried to go home with home healthcare and physical therapy ordered. Unfortunately, she fell again when getting up to go to the bathroom one night. Her daughter called 911 and the patient was readmitted under observation status. Two days later she was transferred to a local rehab facility, where she slowly made a full recovery over the next month. The client contacted us when they received a bill for over $10,000. Medicare had refused to pay because the prior hospitalization had been under observation status.

It is always easier for geriatric care managers or professional advocates to save clients money if we are called in early to oversee the patient's hospitalization. We make sure that the right questions are being asked on the front end so patients and families do not reap serious consequences on the back end when the bills come due. Although we cannot always change the admission status, at least we can ask all the crucial questions that healthcare consumers may not even be aware of, which is a critical task and perk of enlisting the help of a PPHA. Sometimes, a simple coding adjustment can make a critical difference in your medical bills!

*Again, the Tax Cuts and Jobs Act will yield significant changes to the Affordable Care Act. The Congressional Budget Office predicts that this bill will raise insurance premiums even more, and leave more Americans without health insurance. The aftermath of these effects is impossible to know, but for the meantime one thing remains clear; navigating the field of American healthcare remains complex, confusing, and messy.

Understanding Medicare

by Jean Lyon

Ah, Medicare: that magic word! You've finally reached the long-awaited age of sixty-five. And while you're definitely not excited about turning another year older, you *are* definitely excited about one thing: free healthcare insurance!

Or is it?

Sorry to be the bearer of bad news, but **Medicare is NOT FREE!**

Medicare is NOT Medicaid. Before we even get started, let's clarify the terminology (and don't worry: everyone gets these two mixed up). Medicare is the health insurance offered for seniors. Medicaid is public aid, a social healthcare program for families and individuals with low income and limited resources. It doesn't help that the place that runs Medicare also runs Medicaid: CMS, The Centers for Medicare and Medicaid Services. No wonder the two are often confused!

Step one: sign up! There you are: lounging, big smile on your face, your cone-shaped birthday hat firmly in place, stretched out on a footstool – ahh! You happily picture opening your mailbox to see that special birthday present for turning sixty-five... a brand new Medicare card. Uh... think again.

First of all, unless you're already drawing Social Security at age sixty-five, a Medicare card is not going to miraculously appear in your mailbox (sorry). No, you have to be proactive and sign up! You'll have three months before you turn sixty-five, the month of your birthday and three months after you turn sixty-five to sign up for Medicare. This involves either going to medicare.gov, calling Social Security or going to the Social Security office (and a fun way to spend your birthday that is!). And no, it's not like your dentist. You won't receive a friendly reminder notice in the mail that it's time to sign up. You have to do it all on your own.

Medicare only covers the premium for Medicare Part A. While it is true that if you've worked and paid into Social Security for forty quarters (ten years), you will receive Medicare, that is only for the *premium* for Medicare Part A. Here's what no one tells you: *you have to pay for everything else.* You're still on the hook for the deductibles, co-pays, co-insurance and other premiums (more about this later).

All the parts of Medicare. Well, what else is there? Medicare has four parts to it: Medicare Part A (hospital), Medicare Part B (doctors), Medicare Part C (Medicare Advantage, to be discussed later) and Medicare Part D (pharmacy). So while the premium for Medicare Part A is covered, you'll still need to pay the premium for Medicare Part B and Medicare Part D. And, even with these premium payments, this still won't pay for all of your healthcare expenses. The premiums listed will cover only 80% of your medical care; you're liable for the remaining 20% (that 20% is what the insurance types mean by 'co-pay'). In order to help offset the remainder, you're going to also need a Medicare supplement.

The hospital. Let's say you're in the hospital for ten days. Even for a relatively minor issue, that bill would very likely be—at a minimum—in the $50,000 range. If Medicare covered 80%, you would still be liable for $10,000. Gulp. This is where the Medicare Supplements come in. A supplement will often cover approximately 80% of this remaining $10,000, leaving you to pay $2,000. Still a lot, but better than $10,000 and certainly better than shelling out $50,000!

And don't forget the deductible... Before your Medicare Part A hospital coverage kicks in, you'll also have to pay the deductible. While these are not the actual figures, this chapter will utilize ballpark figures. For Medicare Part A, your deductible will be approximately $1,400. Bear in mind, most Medicare supplements will pay part or all of this deductible.

But—please—make sure you're an admitted patient. The first step: make sure that you have been an "admitted patient" and not "under observation." Why? Because Medicare Part A does not go into effect unless you are an admitted patient. Let's say you've taken a nasty fall, you go to an emergency room and you are now under observation. Until you are actually admitted to the hospital, Medicare Part A benefits do not begin. You will need to use your Medicare Part B coverage until you're admitted (more on Medicare Part B later).

Once you are a bona fide admitted patient, your first sixty days in the hospital are covered, and for the majority of people—particularly with the pressure on hospitals to keep patients for as little time as possible — sixty days will usually be enough hospital insurance, unless you have a serious chronic illness.

Rehab facility/skilled nursing. However, it doesn't mean that everything will be covered once you leave the hospital and you need to go to a rehab facility. Remember that "admitted vs. observation" issue?

You need three midnights in the hospital. If, for example, you've had a knee replacement and you need to rehab in a skilled nursing rehab facility, you must have spent at least *three consecutive midnights as an admitted patient* at the hospital for Medicare Part A to cover your rehab stay. If you do not have three consecutive midnights, unless you have additional insurance, you will have to pay privately for your stay at the rehab facility.

Now you get it. You've made sure to stay three consecutive midnights in the hospital. You've discharged from the hospital, transferred to the rehab facility, and you're thinking, *Whew! Thank goodness I skimmed that Medicare chapter! Now Medicare will cover my rehab stay.* Yes and no. Maybe it's time to read a little more carefully…

Medicare only covers the first twenty days in full at the rehab facility. Medicare Part A will cover your first twenty days in full. But after this, for days 21 to 100, Medicare Part A only provides the insured with — using ballpark figures — $175 per day. But OK, you say, that sounds like a lot, isn't that enough? If the daily cost for room and board at the rehab facility is $350 per day (and it's often more), this means you have to pay to the remaining $175 per day. If you were to stay the full 100 days, your share would be $14,000 (80 day x $175). However, if you do have a Medicare supplement, your share will often be reduced to $2,800 — the supplement pays 80% of that remaining fee and you pay 20% of it out-of-pocket.

Also: you have to demonstrate improvement. It can be another story if the patient discharged from the hospital is a frail elderly person or has a form of dementia. In these scenarios, it is challenging for the patient to demonstrate enough improvement to qualify for Medicare Part A. If they cannot follow instructions or they are too weak to actually rehab, the care would not be covered by Medicare.

Let's go into more detail about "nursing home" care. Here's a common scenario. A rushed and harried adult child comes into a retirement community. The adult child, Susie, has picked the most attractive hotel-like place she could find close to her home. And more importantly, based on her research, this retirement place offers excellent care. She then tells the counselor the following story.

On a recent visit to her mother, Susie saw that she was as hale and hearty as always, but when she opened the refrigerator, Susie was horrified to see that her mother had placed her shoes on the top shelf. Worse, Susie then realized her mother placed milk in her bedroom closet. The milk had gone sour and the stench engulfed the entire room. Alarmed, and juggling one hundred other work and home duties, Susie hurriedly researched local retirement communities and made an appointment. This is what brought her to the meeting that morning.

After meeting with the counselor, Susie toured the community, patting herself on the back that she had indeed made an excellent choice. In fact, because her mother is so healthy, she discovers her mother won't even have to move into the skilled nursing area.

The person who gave her the tour informs her that her mother can move to the nice apartments called "Assisted Living Memory Care." Great!

Relieved, Susie pulled out her mother's Medicare card with a flourish, plopped it on the table, and asked to move her mother into the nice apartments right away. The room grew quiet. The counselor had to inform Susie that all of her mother's Assisted Living care is called "custodial care" and it is *not covered by Medicare.*

What? Yes, all custodial care is private pay. "Independent Living," "Assisted Living," and "Memory Care" are not covered by Medicare. Even more painful: most "Skilled Nursing Care" (what most people think of when they think of nursing home care) is not covered by Medicare.

Medicare does not cover custodial care. Medicare only covers "acute care": care for acute events, such as a stroke, a fall, a heart attack, etc. Unfortunately, Medicare does not pay for long-term care resulting from a chronic medical condition. When you consider that Independent Living up to Skilled Nursing care can cost between $50,000 to $100,000 respectively or more per year, this is a sobering thought.

Medicare Part B (doctor). So, what is this Medicare B all about? Medicare B is insurance for doctor's visits and lab work. And unlike Medicare Part A, for Medicare Part B, you have to pay a monthly premium. The amount can vary depending on your income. However, again using approximate figures, the premium would be roughly $150 per month or $1,800 per year. In addition, there is a deductible, approximately of $200. After this, your doctor's visits, etc. would be covered 80% and you would be responsible for the remaining 20%. Again, you would need a supplement policy to cover the bulk of the remaining charges.

Medicare Part D (pharmacy). While most people are aware — or at least have heard of — Medicare Part B, a surprisingly large number of people are not aware of Medicare Part D, nor do they sign up for it. Is this really that big of deal? Yes! You'll see why in a minute.

As with Medicare Part B, Medicare Part D entails an initial deductible. You can count on a deductible of around $425. After that, you're responsible for your monthly premium. Without getting into too much detail, Medicare A and Medicare B are called "Original Medicare" and they are managed by the federal government. On the other hand, Medicare Part D is managed by private insurance companies. Because of this, the premiums can vary greatly. But on average, the premium would be approximately $50 per month or $480 per year.

You're now aware of Medicare Part D, but you say to yourself, hey, I only use one cholesterol med and it only costs about $10 a month. Why on earth should I pay an additional $50 per month?

Good question. Yes, that's what you pay now. But let's say three years down the road you (God forbid) have a major health catastrophe. You discharge from the hospital, but instead of your measly $10 monthly pharmacy bill, you are suddenly saddled with a whopping $1,600 monthly pharmacy bill (and this is not pie-in-the-sky, this sort of amount is sadly common after an acute medical event). So now, because you do have Medicare Part D — which is normally split 75% paid by the insurance company and your responsibility of 25% — your share of this pharmacy bill is $400 instead of the $1,600. Over the course of a year, if you're required to continue taking these meds each month, that would amount to well over a $14,000 savings for prescriptions alone.

Aha! You think, well, if that's the case, I'll just sign up for Medicare Part D when I do have these mammoth pharmacy bills. Not so fast. Medicare is way ahead of you.

Late enrollment penalties. Like any other type of insurance, Medicare operates under the premise of everyone pooling their resources together and those pooled resources offset the care of the people drawing from the combined funds. In essence, Medicare relies on everyone signing up as soon as they are eligible. The good news? At age sixty-five, no one can be underwritten. That means everyone qualifies for Medicare, no matter what their state of health may be. On the other hand, as part of this deal, Medicare is banking on many healthy individuals signing up at age sixty-five. If everyone just waited to sign up when they needed intense pharmacy or medical attention, it would unfairly place the burden on those who did sign up on time. The system would not work.

But no problem if you're sixty-five, working, and you have insurance. To clarify, if you are sixty-five or older, still employed (at a company with twenty or more employees), and you have credible health insurance (not COBRA!), you do not have to sign up for Medicare yet. You can continue using your company's insurance or decide if you wish to receive Medicare Part A as a supplement to your current health insurance (since it won't cost you anything) and wait to enroll in Medicare Part B once you retire.

Medicare Part B: late enrollment penalties. To combat people waiting to enroll until they're sick and need the coverage, Medicare has late enrollment penalties for people who sign up late. For Medicare Part B, that penalty is 10% for every 12-month period you didn't sign up. In this case, if you signed up three years late (it can happen…), the $150 monthly premium rises to $150 x 10%=$15. $15 penalty x 3=$45. You think, well, big deal, $45-I'll pay that! Let's clarify, that's $150 (base fee) + $45 (penalty) =$195 per month, not a one-time fee. You still think, well, OK, that's not great, but I'll just repay that amount for the next three years. Here's the newsflash-that penalty is permanent. Instead of paying $150 per month, you're stuck with $195… forever. Not that this amount will be fixed. The base amount increases every year, so the base and penalty would increase every year. Moral of the story: sign up on time.

Medicare Part D: late enrollment penalties. Now let's look at the far more common occurrence: people signing up late for Medicare Part D. Because the monthly premiums are based on the open market, the calculation is a little more nebulous. The calculation is 1% of the average fee x the number of months. If Medicare deems the monthly average premium to be $50, the 1% amounts to 50 cents. Now you're really thinking, *phtt!* Ding me with the 50 cents, who cares? But again, that average fee is multiplied by the number of months, i.e. 50 cents for one year =$6. But if you're three years late, $6 x 3=$18. You're still thinking, OK, eighteen bucks — ha! I'll pay it. Again, Medicare is not saying this will be a one-time penalty of $18. No, that fee is added to your monthly premium; $50 + $18=$68, every month for as long as you use Medicare. And, just like with Medicare Part B, the base fee increases each year.

But — caveat — in both instances, with Medicare Part B or Medicare Part D, even if you were misinformed, didn't quite understand about the deadline, or you were rolling the dice, hoping you didn't need the insurance — and now you find you'll be dinged with a penalty... sign up anyway! Yes, it would not be pleasant to have to pay, let's say, 25% or 30% more for the premium, but it's a pittance compared to paying those future healthcare expenses out-of-pocket.

The Donut Hole. I would be remiss not to mention the infamous Donut Hole. This used to be a much bigger problem because the size of the donut hole used to be much bigger. The term refers to a coverage gap for Medicare Part D. Until your drug expenses reach a certain amount within the year (around $4,000) insurance pays roughly 75% of the bill, you pay 25%. After this point, you are in... the Donut Hole! (Cue scary music.) Not long ago, once you were in the coverage gap, insurance paid for nothing until your pharmacy bills reached an amount Medicare D calls "Catastrophic Coverage."

But nowadays, insurance pays for approximately 50% of this "coverage gap" until the insured's expenses reach the "Catastrophic Coverage" amount of around $5,000. In other words, $5,000 -$4,000=$1,000 — there is a gap of $1,000. Instead of Medicare Part D paying 75% of this amount, it pays approximately 50% of charges (and it will depend on the 'tiers' of drugs used). So instead of paying your normal share of $250 for this amount, you're liable for $500 while in the Donut Hole. Medicare is filling this hole at a rate of 10% per year and this gap is slated to be filled by the year 2020. No more donuts!

Medicare Part C. And what was that Medicare Part C that was mentioned before? Medicare Part C replaces Original Medicare. With Original Medicare, you would have Medicare Part A and Part B with a Medicare Part D policy added to it and a Medigap supplement (got it? Easy peasy, right?). Medicare Part C, known as Medicare Advantage, bundles them all into one. To be clear, you still would need to pay your Medicare Part B premium, but Medicare Part C replaces Part A and Part B, and includes Part D. You would not need to buy separate supplement or pharmacy insurance.

But why would you want to do that? For a couple of reasons. Mostly, your personal preference. Original Medicare + Medicare Part D pharmacy coverage offers you more choices. In essence, although not all Medigap policies work this way, you're able to go to any hospital or doctor who accepts Medicare. Pretty nice! But you do pay for it. While the flexibility can be a convenient option, you pay for that Medigap policy whether you use it or not.

A Medicare Advantage policy, on the other hand, operates more like an HMO or a PPO (Medicare Part C offers both of these options as well as some additional specialty plans). In the positive column, although you are restricted to a particular network, the networks are large and you often pay a low premium or no premium at all. But in the negative column, if you don't live in a large urban area, there can be higher initial deductibles. And to confuse matters more, Medigap policies have to be chosen carefully because some Medigap policies do not have a Maximum Out-of-Pocket cap. All Medicare Advantage plans offer this cap. Again, it's all about your personal preference and level of comfort.

What Medicare doesn't cover at all. Here's something that comes as a surprise to many people transitioning into Medicare, there are several key things that Medicare doesn't cover at all. No vision. Medicare does not pay for optometry visits or glasses. No dental. Medicare does not pay for dental visits or dentures. No hearing. Medicare does not pay for hearing tests or — more importantly — hearing aids (which can be very pricey). Some

Medicare advantage policies do cover all or part of these.

Medicare Election times. No, no, you're not casting a vote. You're making your Medicare choices and you can't do this any old time. There are basically four times you can make your election:

1. **Initial Enrollment Period**

   - 3 months before you turn 65
   - The month of your birthday
   - 3 months after you turn 65
   - 7 months total

And the great news about this Initial Enrollment Period: as detailed before, you cannot be disqualified for pre-existing conditions.

What if you miss these deadlines?

2. **General Enrollment Period**

   - January 1 to March 31
   - Coverage begins July 1st

You use this time to sign up for Medicare Part A and Part B... but not Part D. If you enroll late for Part D, you'll have to wait for Special Enrollment (April 1 to June 30) or for Open Enrollment (isn't this fun?).

3. **Open Enrollment Period** (also called **Annual Enrollment Period**)

   - Oct. 15th to Dec. 7th
   - "Preview" begins October 1st

Open Enrollment is set at the end of the year to review price increases for the upcoming year. This is the time actually allotted for Medicare users to opt in to Medicare Advantage, Medicare Part C. But, it can be used for other things too. So even if you're not opting to change to Medicare Part C, you might want to use this time to see if your plan (Medigap or Medicare Advantage) will increase beginning in the upcoming year. During Open Enrollment, you could then switch to a more economical plan. Or let's say during the course of the year, your doctor has prescribed more medications than you used to take. You could take advantage of the Open Enrollment time to determine if a different Medicare Part D prescription plan will offer lower prices for the new meds you now use.

Overall, Open Enrollment is a perfect time to either change from Medigap to Medicare Advantage, to find out if your current Medigap or Medicare Advantage plan will increase in price and find a comparable plan that might be less expensive or to see if a different Medicare Part D plan offers lower prices on the meds you use. This is an ideal time to review your plans and change them if you want. That's what all the hoopla is all about!

4. Special Enrollment can happen any time... it's Special!

- It can happen if someone worked past sixty-five, has now retired and wants to enroll in Medicare Part B, Medicare Part D and a Medicare supplement

- Or if someone moves to a different area and they want to change plans.

And remember, if you worked past sixty-five, you have eight months from the time your health insurance or employment ends (important: this does not include COBRA!). But this Special

Enrollment period can be important for everyone.

Why? Because any time you (or a loved one) moves temporarily or permanently to a skilled nursing facility, this also counts as a 'move.' Everyone seems to overlook this key fact. Therefore, you qualify for Special Election and you can change your Medicare coverage. If you are making a move to a skilled facility, this is an excellent time to review your supplemental plans and possibly change them. Often, the individual's care has become more critical and a different plan may be more beneficial.

Review your coverage every year. Annual review of your Medicare insurance and review after an acute event cannot be emphasized enough. Many, many seniors who have Medicare just made one decision when they turned sixty-five and they never looked at their plan again, sticking with the same old tried-and-true plan through the years. This can be a very costly mistake! If you feel daunted at the prospect of analyzing your Medicare plan again, ask your insurance professional — or you can have your fourteen-year-old grandson pull up a comparison on their computer, iPad, smartphone, or whatever else they'll be using soon.

At this point, you think, let me get this straight. That Medicare card only covers the Medicare Part A premium. I'm on the hook for the premium for Medicare Part B, Medicare Part D, and my Medicare supplement insurance. And even with all of this, if I need long-term care, most of that is private pay? Yes. That's the bottom line.

Are there any options? Well, yes. The truth is that the bulk of your healthcare expenses will occur towards the end of your life. And, financial experts calculate that Medicare only covers approximately 12% of this end-of-life care. Other than just paying out-of-pocket, there are a few options.

- **Supportive Living Facility (SLF).** If the senior only needs Assisted Living, there is the alternative available of a Supportive Living Facility. The government pays a portion of the care if the senior meets certain income requirements.

- **Long-term care insurance.** Depending on the policy, if a senior has a long-term care insurance policy, they can use its benefits to help defray the cost of home health care, assisted living and skilled nursing. This will normally pay for a substantial portion of their care.

Now, now, no rolling of the eyes when long-term care insurance is mentioned. Times have changed! Long-term care insurance policies have evolved and there are many more 'hybrid' options of long-term care insurance combined with more familiar life insurance products. Also, there are now more embedded safeguards with inflation protection and tax qualified policies where a portion of the premium is not taxed. In addition, with the newer hybrid plans, if you don't end up needing the long-term care insurance, you do not lose what you've paid into it.

- Medicaid. The senior can go on a "spend down" to qualify for Medicaid (public aid). You think, go ahead and switch me to Medicaid, let the government pay! I'll just move my assets over to my kids (and hope they don't spend it all..), and then the government will pay for the nursing home expense. Er, sorry, but the government does a five-year "look back" to see if the senior's assets have been moved.

Plan. Ideally, it's far better for the family to meet with a financial advisor when the senior is younger, healthier, and not in a moment of crisis to devise a financial plan for their long-term care. And, by the way, this includes choosing a durable Power of Attorney for Healthcare and for Finance (Property). It's better for checks and balances (pardon the pun) for two separate people to have these roles. If you're unable to speak for yourself, you need to have someone you trust do this for you!

So now you've pulled off your birthday party hat and you're sitting up straight, stunned, absorbing the news. But it's not all bad. And yes, the sad truth is that Medicare is not free. But the good news is that Medicare is still statistically much less expensive than the majority of commercial healthcare insurance plans. With a little foresight and planning, you can optimize your coverage and plan to make your senior years as sunny and relaxing as possible.

Jean Lyon, MBA, is the owner of Lyon Retirement Solutions, www.lyonretirementsolutions.com, an insurance company dedicated to Medicare insurance. With her extensive background in the senior care and the pharmacy industries, she consults seniors and adult children on their various Medicare choices; tailoring their needs during Open Enrollment, saving money during annual reviews and assisting with long-term care planning.

For detailed information, please contact Medicare or refer to your Medicare & You Medicare Handbook. This information is educational in nature regarding senior citizen's healthcare and Medicare coverage and services. Information contained in this chapter is general in nature, it is not meant to replace the advice of healthcare professionals. If you have specific healthcare needs, or for complete information, please see a doctor or other healthcare provider. Although the author has made every effort to ensure the contents of this information are correct and complete, the author cannot be held responsible for the accuracy of information. Information on Medicare parts and policies may contain inaccuracies, errors or can be changed or updated without notice and therefore may be out of date. This is not a complete listing of plans available in your service area. For a complete listing please contact 1-800-MEDICARE (TTY users should call 1-877-486-2048), 24 hours a day/7 days a week or consult www.medicare.gov.

People ask me all the time what I think of the Affordable Care Act overall. I must preface my comments first by saying that I have a unique vantage point; most of our clients come to us because they are unhappy with some aspect of modern healthcare, and we fight for them. Families and patients are either frightened, angry, lost, or confused, and they hire us to untangle messes and protect their loved ones.

And for many people, there is very little that is affordable about the Affordable Care Act (ACA, or Obamacare). We get calls every week from people who are frustrated with higher insurance premiums and continuing rising costs of healthcare. Though it is true that ACA-compliant insurance plans must now cover prevention services at no cost to the consumer, as well as emergency medical services, some customers are frustrated at the rising deductibles that are necessary for affordable insurance premiums. Whether or not all ER visits are covered by insurance is a matter of open debate, as the client usually has out-of-pocket expenses due to higher deductibles necessary for affordable premiums.

Our company does many public service education programs that empower the general public. Education is power. Current information about the rapidly changing healthcare environment in our country is important for all consumers. As we age, the chances grow that we will one day be admitted to a hospital. People in crisis do not learn well. Anxiety and stress affect how we process information. It is best to become knowledgeable about navigating healthcare challenges before the crisis occurs.

Another challenge for seniors is to find good supplemental plans to their Medicare policies (as discussed in the *Intricacies of Medicare* chapter). Many expensive medications are coming off insurance formularies due to Medicare cost containment. Some of these medicines are critical to those with neurological diseases or undergoing chemotherapy. It is important to have a trusted professional to help weed through the many plans and help consumers choose the right plan for their specific needs. The industry is growing more complex every day and it is hard for the average layperson to know which plan is best for their needs. Often, insurance brokers will sell plans that they get the highest sales commissions for. Spending the money today to hire an advocate who will research your best options can save you tens of thousands of dollars in the future.

Disabled people are disproportionately affected by these challenges as well. This makes me angry because they need our country's help the most, as do the elderly, the poor, and those struggling with mental illness. Many cannot work and live with serious limitations, be they physical, emotional, or cognitive. Unless they are wealthy, they cannot afford the massive costs associated with their disability. The system is set up to control costs and does not always persevere with individuals for the long run. William's story, in an earlier chapter, illustrated this perfectly.

I am sincerely concerned about how these new policies hurt our seniors and result in frustrated healthcare workers who are pushed harder and harder to document more, move along faster than ever, and watch the bottom line above all. From what I have seen, business and medicine do not always mix well.

You know your own healthcare spending, but what does the utilization of those dollars look like across the rest of the country? A recent study done by the Dartmouth Institute for Health Policy included a national atlas showing great variations in healthcare cost and utilization (Dartmouthatlas.org). Atul Gwande, the physician who wrote the groundbreaking book, 'Being Mortal' in 2014, agrees with many of the conclusions of the Dartmouth study.

There is a wide variation in how money on healthcare is spent in different areas of our country. In population-dense locations where affluence is present, the culture of money encourages physicians and hospitals to order, spend, and use more product than in low-income areas. Healthcare waste and fraud is a massive problem in our country, and government restrictions imposed by the Affordable Care Act have done little to rein in costs. Many consumers have noted rising costs of insurance, higher out-of-pocket expenses, and higher hospital bills since 2010 when the ACA was signed into law.

After reviewing the Dartmouth Atlas, several things are apparent to me. First: there is a wide variation in the numbers of seniors who live in different parts of the country. As a general rule, the north and the east coast have a greater percentage of people 75 or older. Generally, fewer seniors want to live in the southwest and Alaska. Second: poverty levels vary greatly in different regions. Older poor people are sicker and utilize more healthcare dollars when they do enter the system. It is what it is.

I believe different utilization patterns are also dependent upon how physicians practice in different regions. Studies now show that primary care physicians are the best at keeping patients out of hospitals. Most hospitals today use hospitalists to care for inpatients, discouraging primary care physicians from continuing to care for their patients when they enter the institution. Only 50 percent of people nationally have a primary care physician, and often depend upon emergency rooms for acute illnesses. Emergency rooms are the most expensive places of all to receive healthcare.

Patient culture also factors into utilization. Proximity to hospitals, disease burden, education, race, and economy all play a role. It has long been known that older African-Americans have a general distrust of the American healthcare system, and often hide their illnesses and refuse to get early intervention for health problems. Diseases like diabetes and hypertension have a higher prevalence in the African-American community as well, and have serious consequences if left untreated.

Another problem in utilization of healthcare may be related to Medicare itself. While commercial insurance companies incentivize healthcare consumers to live healthy lifestyles with lower insurance premiums for quitting smoking, losing weight, and undergoing yearly health assessments, Medicare has no such watchdog programs built in. In fact, slightly over 10 percent of Medicare recipients nationally take advantage of yearly free health checkups with their doctors.

A few words now about legal healthcare documents. No one likes to talk about them, but everyone needs them. The most difficult, but vitally necessary, legal forms that all adults over 18 should have is a healthcare power of attorney.

A healthcare power of attorney names a surrogate decision-maker who can step in and make healthcare decisions on a person's behalf. It is a more legal and binding document than a living will, and it is the one that hospitals always ask for when a person arrives at the hospital in an unconscious state. A person must be mentally competent to assign another person rights to act as a healthcare power of attorney. If the senior becomes mentally incompetent or unable to make their own decisions, due to a stroke, dementia, or any condition that renders them unconscious, the family will need to go to court to have a legal guardian assigned. This can be costly and time-consuming. Capacity vs. competence is a big topic that your PPHA or attorney can inform you more about. Try to avoid guardianship and probate if you can; it is time-consuming, costly, and difficult. In most cases, a POA (power of attorney) for health and estate can help you avoid these extreme measures.

In the absence of a POA for healthcare in place, hospitals may ask the family to assign a family member "surrogate decision-maker" status, but for long-term decisions, a guardianship procedure will be necessary for patients who do not have a healthcare power of attorney documented. The form can be easily obtained on each state government's website and usually does not need to be notarized. Families can do the documentation themselves, but it is wise to have a healthcare professional or attorney assist them, in case the issue of competence should be questioned by anyone at a later time. Financial/household power-of-attorney designation should always be done with an attorney present, as is true with wills and trusts. If a person dies without a will or trust, the person's estate will be dispersed by the probate court. Going through probate is—again—time-consuming and expensive, as the court takes a percentage of the estate's value for court costs. Planning ahead will avoid frustration and save time and money for all concerned.

There are other ethical dilemmas out there in this shifting healthcare landscape that concern me. One controversial law, already adopted in many states, is called the POLST (Physician Order for Life-Sustaining Treatment). It replaces the old Do Not Resuscitate (DNR) order that families and physicians would sign when they determined that heroic measures would no longer be used if the patient stopped breathing or had a cardiac arrest. The POLST law adds some new caveats that some people feel give physicians too much control in life-or-death situations. I learned this in the case of a young woman I will call Wu-Lin.

Wu-Lin and her husband were both doctoral students at a large university on the near north side of Chicago. They were delighted when Wu-Lin became pregnant with their first child, a son. This would be the first grandson on both sides of the family, and their parents and Wu-Lin's brother were all in China awaiting the happy event.

One morning, Wu-Lin woke up with a severe headache. It progressed and caused sensitivity to light, nausea, and vomiting. Her husband rushed her to the local emergency room, where the doctors saw signs that indicated an intra-cranial bleed, so they ordered a stat MRI scam. While Wu-Lin was in the MRI room, she started seizing and a code blue was called. She had developed an intra-cranial hemorrhage from a small aneurysm, stressed by the increased circulating blood volume of pregnancy. She was 28 years old and eight months pregnant.

Physicians rushed to MRI and put her on life support, performed a crash C-section (saving the baby boy), inserted an intra-ventricular drain in her skull to relieve the pressure and evacuate the blood, and sent her to ICU. When frantic family members contacted me two days later, it was because doctors were telling, not asking, the family that life support would be removed the following day.

When I walked into her room in the ICU that afternoon, I could see signs of brain death: fixed, dilated pupils; copious amounts of urine draining from her catheter (diabetes insipidus occurs when the mid-brain is damaged and the body loses its ability to regulate fluids properly); high doses of three vasopressors; very fast heart rate; very low blood pressure. After confirming the doctor's report that she appeared to be brain-dead, I spent time with the family and listened to the devastation they were going through.

The mother of this beautiful young woman was concerned about getting her son to the U.S. before she died; the doctors were pushing hard to have Wu-Lin's life support removed before her brother could get his emergency visa and fly into Chicago-O'Hare the following day. In the Dhao religion, if a person dies on the wrong day of the Chinese calendar, they will not be reunited with their ancestors. This was important to the family; Wu-Lin should die on a good day.

That evening, we convened with the family at a patient care conference. Wu-Lin's grieving family and the doctors assigned to her case met for several hours to try and reach a resolution. The doctors told them that since she had been declared brain-dead, they did not need permission to remove her life support. And technically, they were right. The POLST law makes it clear that once someone has been declared brain-dead, they are legally dead.

I had never personally seen doctors use that prerogative in a case such as this. The neurosurgeon on Wu-Lin's case was particularly abrasive and insensitive to the grieving family. At one point, the mother of the dying woman threw herself down upon the carpet and sobbed hysterically.

I stopped the meeting and requested a full ethics committee meeting to evaluate the case the following day.

Hospitals don't like it when outsiders request an ethics committee hearing. It means that community members who sit on the committee will hear the hospital's dirty laundry aired publicly. It means that someone on the outside questions the ethics and integrity of the hospital. It's embarrassing. This is probably why the hospital staff in William's story did not invite the community members of the ethics committee to his hearing.

The following day, nearly two dozen of us crowded into a hospital conference room to hear from the family. Through a Mandarin interpreter, they poignantly described to us who Wu-Lin was: a brilliant scholar, a beautiful young woman filled with hope, someone with a bright future. She was a loving wife, a kind and tender mother-to-be.

The family told a much more difficult story as well: one of cold, stern, and uncompromising physicians who exhibited no sensitivity for what the family was going through. I looked around the room as ethics committee members grew shocked and sad. When the doctors were mentioned, people looked down at their hands or turned away, sometimes with tears in their eyes. Wu-Lin's husband looked into my eyes the entire time he spoke, and told me afterward that my face gave him courage to go on. He and his mother-in-law embraced me and offered their thanks for standing by them and giving them courage as they spoke.

I will never know why the doctors were so insistent on being the ones to determine the hour of Wu-Lin's death. The ICU had six empty beds that day; I cannot imagine what the rush was. The ethics committee suggested that they allow the family the extra time they requested for Wu-Lin's brother to arrive. Instead, the doctors removed her life support one hour before his plane landed the following day.

I don't know if money played a role in this case or not, but I do know that hospitals are under pressure to contain costs and justify utilization of healthcare dollars. Who knows? It may simply have been a control issue.

Wu-Lin's husband ultimately went back to China with his parents and in-laws. They are helping him raise his son, whose name means "happy" in Mandarin.

Tips to Equip: Getting your documents in order

1. **Assign a healthcare power of attorney** to make those decisions on your behalf should you become incapacitated.

2. **Separately, if possible, assign a financial POA with an attorney present.** If you die without a will, your estate could be held up for years in probate court. Not only will this be costly and time consuming for the loved ones you've left behind, the court takes a piece of your estate in addition to deciding how it will be dispersed between your family.

3. **Check into your state's laws regarding Do Not Resuscitate orders**; they may have changed to empower physicians to enact the new POLST order. This gives physicians more

power than your family to decide when you legally die. Know your rights under your state's law.

Conclusion
It All Points to This...

By now, you've learned just how crucial the task of advocating for yourself or your loved one is to the quality of your life, your health, and your rights. This book is a valuable tool-kit to patients and families everywhere, a manual to become an active participant and an informed healthcare consumer who will not settle for anything less than safe, high-quality medical care.

My colleagues and I have covered the gamut: what it means to be an advocate; all of the different considerations at stake, such as legal documents; alternate means of treatment; and your rights under various circumstances, as well as how to exert them. Now you can protect yourself in different situations; whether that is your person, your safety or your belongings. Now you know who can benefit from having an advocate, which is the easiest question to answer of them all: anyone who is a healthcare recipient can benefit from having an advocate on their side!

You understand what it takes to be an advocate, as well as the different types of advocates available; and which type of advocate has the most resources at their disposal to solve complex problems (which I firmly believe will always be the nurse advocate; our far-reaching background, our variety of specialties, situations, and challenges we've faced throughout our clinical careers make us the ideal healthcare advocates!).

I will reiterate: there are many types of advocates. Hopefully, I've provided enough information and tips to equip, educate, and empower you to help you do your due diligence. If you decide an advocate is the right way to go for your unique situation, you now have the know-how at your disposal to choose the best fit.

I would be remiss to end this extensive collection of valuable tips and information without summarizing how effective a champion nurse advocate can be, least of all for the perks we provide.

Depending on the situation, a nurse advocate, who is medically trained, can put together a complete medical profile for you that is worth its weight in gold. This can be especially helpful if you're seeing multiple physicians, or if you make unscheduled trips to the ER, as a way to improve communication between physicians. Communication is paramount where life-saving decisions are concerned. And depending on how savvy you are, the complete medical profile may cover the extent of what you may need to carry forward on your own!

I have endeavored most of all to leave you with this: I and my colleagues are more concerned now than ever for patients trying to keep up with constant changes in healthcare. We all require the ability to navigate it successfully and have positive outcomes. And in today's miasma of information, I am concerned for the safety of all healthcare recipients.

Even though nurses and physicians are doing the very best they can to give high-quality, safe, and efficient care with the increased demands of the post-ACA healthcare economy, we also know — in a way that only clinicians can — how the system can fail patients. Hospital-based physicians and nurses everywhere will tell you: never ins US history has the need for patient advocacy been greater.

My ultimate hope for this book is that it will in some way help on a wider scale—more healthcare recipients than I can ever hope to reach patient-to-patient—since it is impossible to save every single person who could benefit from the resources at my disposal.

While I know it will likely take a long time to fix our broken healthcare system, we, as patients and the loved ones of patients, must advocate for ourselves. And if we cannot, we must find someone who knows how to advocate for us. A private professional healthcare advocate is someone you should ideally have on speed dial, but barring that, I pray this book may serve a multitude of patients that may not be able to hire one.

Why Nurses (and Patient Advocacy, in general) Matter

This past week, I had a uniquely memorable and inspiring experience. I was invited to speak about my career path and the role I play as a private professional RN patient advocate. When I arrived at the venue, a small classroom lab at the College of Lake County was packed with about 50 nursing students, many of them getting ready to graduate in three months and enter the work force. They wanted to know what was "around the bend" and what they could expect when they entered the real world of modern day healthcare. Several other seasoned nurses from various specialties were there and gave testimonies and advice for student nurses getting ready to take the big exam and get ready for their first interviews.

I was inspired, humbled and excited for them. I looked into their eyes and saw the excitement and nervousness, the eagerness to go out and make a difference in the world. And I thought "How lucky I am to have chosen to be a nurse!" Today being a hospital nurse is in many ways more difficult than it was when

I graduated. In 1976, nurses were taught to spend time with their patients, develop thorough teaching plans and hone our assessment skills, as we who spend the most time with patients were often the one to pick up a small change that could lead to a catastrophic event in the hospital. One of my most memorable instructors was an old Army nurse who took no nonsense from any of us. She would walk us into a patient's room, let us stand there for two minutes and notice as many things as we could about the room, the patient and the environment and walk out. We then had a contest: who would be able to make note of and remember the most things accurately and record them on a paper afterward. The student who noticed the most about the room and patient would win that day. The point she was making was that we first develop the observation skills, then put them into a critical judgement/observation practice that would save lives and influence treatment when we knew what kinds of assessment changes the doctor would need to know about quickly.

We are the doctor's eyes and ears when they're not there and doctors depend upon good nursing to prevent harm. Today many of those skills are being lost for nurses who are taught that documentation is everything; if it's not charted, it did not happen, etc. Two thirds of nurses' time must be spent on the computer, and they and their physician colleagues are not happy about it. It is what it is in the modern world of healthcare. And the sad truth is that most practitioners do not have the time to read all that charting anyway. More patient care is done today by unskilled PCT's who focus on tasks; nurses are there to give medications and do brief assessments once or twice per day, or to change wound dressings. But nursing remains in my mind, the most noble, highest calling of any profession I can imagine. Patient advocacy is at the very core of what every good nurse does, day in and day out.

We heal, we comfort, we treat conditions and help mend broken hearts. Does it hurt sometimes? Absolutely…but then there is the joy, the peace that comes from knowing that we make a difference every single day we go to work. And we can change our specialty when we feel burnout coming on in the one we are in. I am a rare 39-year veteran of ICU nursing and I loved it so much…countless cards, emails and memories of thankful patients who told me I saved their loved ones' lives, all give me strength for the battles I face today as a professional advocate. Those shining faces of student nurses earlier this week really touched my heart. The advice I gave them in the end was simple: "Don't you ever let anyone tell you that the computer is more important than the patient! It never will be; every day you have a choice: to take the time to listen, to go out of your way to bring comfort and healing, to go the extra mile to make sure your patient gets superior care. Be courageous. Nurses make the difference. We are the ones who bring the CARE to healthcare: go out and change the world!"

Dear readers,

If you have persevered to the very end of this book, my intention has not been to frighten, discourage, or overwhelm any of you. My aim has been to tell some difficult truths about the real world of modern day healthcare in America. Every doctor and nurse working in hospitals today will tell you that the system is getting less patient centric and more frustrating for all who work in health care. Has healthcare in America become any safer since 1999? The sad truth is no. Multiple studies will show you the facts. We still have medical error as the 3rd leading cause of death in America. It's a fact. So, arm yourself with tools that can help keep you and your loved ones safer. Try to stay out of the hospital by practicing good health habits. Notice little things you've never noticed before. Speak up, ask questions, and proceed with caution. No matter what, everyone today needs their own healthcare advocate.

References

- American Hospital Association. https://www.aha.org.

- Alliance of Professional Health Advocates. (2016). About APHA. Retrieved June 20, 2016, from aphaadvocates. org: www.aphaadvocates.org/about-apha/

- Alzheimer's Association. (n.d.). 2015 Alzheimer's Disease Facts and Figures. Retrieved from alz.org: https:// www.alz.org/facts/downloads/facts_figures_2015. pdfhttps://www.alz.org/facts/downloads/facts_ figures_2015.pdf

- Alzheimers Association. (2016). Residential Care. Retrieved July 8, 2016, from alz.org: http://www.alz. org/care/alzheimers-dementia-residential-facilities. asp#types

- American Geriatric Society. (n.d.). Identifying Medications that Older Adults Should Avoid or Use With Caution: the 2012 American Geriatrics Society Updated Beers Criteria. Retrieved from americangeriatrics.org: http://www.americangeriatrics.org/files/documents/ beers/BeersCriteriaPublicTranslation.pdf

- American Hospital Association. (n.d.). Patient Care Partnership. Retrieved from aha.org: www.aha.org/ content/00-10/pcp_english_030730.pdf

- Andrews, L. B., Stocking, C., & Krizek, T. (1997). An Alternative Method for Studying Adverse Events in Medical Care. Lancet , 349, 309-313.

- Beckers Hospital Review. (2016). 10 Top Patient Safety Issues For 2016. Retrieved from www.beckershospitalreview.com: http://www.beckershospitalreview.com/quality/10-top-patient-safety-issues-for-2016.htmlhttp://www.beckershospitalreview.com/quality/10-top-patient-safety-issues-for-2016.html

- Bureau of Labor Statistics. (2015, May). 29-1126 Respiratory Therapist. Retrieved June 27, 2016, from bls.gov: http://www.bls.gov/oes/current/oes291126.htm

- Cancer Centers Of America. https://www.cancercenter.com

- CBS News. (2017, August). Shortage of primary care physicians could threaten patient care. Retrieved November 11, 2017. https://www.cbsnews.com/news/shortage-of-primary-care-physicians-could-threaten-patient-care/

- Centers for Disease Control and Prevention. (n.d.). Hand Hygiene. Retrieved June 21, 2016, from www.cdc.gov: https://www.cdc.gov/HandHygiene/download/hand_hygiene_core.pdf

- Centers for Disease Control and Prevention. (2016, April 28). Hand Hygiene in Healthcare Settings. Retrieved May 27, 2016, from www.cdc.gov.

- Centers for Disease Control and Prevention. (2016, March 3). Making Healthcare Safer. Retrieved June 1, 2016, from www.cdc.gov: www.cdc.gov/vitalsigns/protect-patients/

- Centers for Disease Control. (2016, March 31). cdc.

gov. Retrieved April 20, 2016, from Autism Spectrum Disorder: http://www.cdc.gov/ncbddd/autism/data.html

- Dartmouth Atlas. http://www.Dartmouthatlas.org

- Gallup. (2014, December 18). Americans Rate Nurses Highest on Honesty, Ethical Standards. Retrieved June 11, 2016, from gallup.com: http://www.gallup.com/poll/180260/americans-rate-nurses-highest-honesty-ethical-standards.aspx

- Institute for Safe Medicine Practices. (2015). ISMP's list of confused drug names. Retrieved June 12, 2016, from ismp.org: http://www.ismp.org/Tools/confuseddrugnames.pdf

- Japsen, B. (2016, March 6). Retrieved May 27, 2016, from www.forbes.com: http://www.forbes.com/sites/brucejapsen/2016/03/06/states-remove-barriers-to-physician-assistants/#60b5583314e7

- Jauhar, S. (2014, August 29). Why Doctors Are Sick Of Their Profession. Retrieved June 4, 2016, from www.wsj.com: http://www.wsj.com/articles/the-u-s-s-ailing-medical-system-a-doctors-perspective-1409325361

- John T. James, P. (2014). A New, Evidence-Based Estimate Of Patient Harms Associated With Hospital Care. Journal of Patient Safety , 9 (3), 122-128.

- Linda T. Kohn, J. M. (2000). To err is human: building a safer health system. National Academy of Sciences. Washington DC: National Academy Press.

- Medicare. (n.d.). Skilled Nursing Facility Checklist. Retrieved from medicare.gov: https://www.medicare.

gov/files/skilled-nursing-facility-checklist.pdf

- Met Life Market Institute. (2011). Market Survey of Long-Term Care Costs: The 2011 MetLife Market Survey of Nursing Home, Assisted Living, Adult Day Services, and Home Care Costs. New York: Metropolitan Life Insurance Company.

- NAHAC. (2015). History of NAHAC. Retrieved June 25, 2016, from www.nahac.memberlodge.com: www.nahac.memberlodge.com/history

- NAHAC. (2015). www.nahac.memberlodge.com. Retrieved June 25, 2016, from http://nahac.memberlodge.com

- National Association of Orthopedic Technologists. (2013). What is an orthopedic technologist? Retrieved July 1, 2016, from naot.org: http://www.naot.org/sections/about.orthotics.php

- Patient Advocate Certification Board. (n.d.). Patient Advocacy vs. Medical Advocacy: View from the PACB. Retrieved from pacboard.org: http://pacboard.org/2016/03/09/patient-advocacy-vs-medical-advocacy-view-from-the-pacb/

- Pew Research Center. (2013). The Sandwich Generation. Retrieved March 20, 2016, from pewsocialtrends.org: http://www.pewsocialtrends.org/2013/01/30/the-sandwich-generation/

Index

CPSIA information can be obtained
at www.ICGtesting.com
Printed in the USA
FFHW021510051119
55952465-61794FF